Information Circular 9506

Guidelines for Permitting, Construction, and Monitoring of Retention Bulkheads in Underground Coal Mines

By Samuel P. Harteis, P.E., Dennis R. Dolinar, and Terence M. Taylor, P.E.

DEPARTMENT OF HEALTH AND HUMAN SERVICES
Centers for Disease Control and Prevention
National Institute for Occupational Safety and Health
Pittsburgh Research Laboratory
Pittsburgh, PA

June 2008

Disclaimer

Mention of any company or product does not constitute endorsement by the National Institute for Occupational Safety and Health (NIOSH). In addition, citations to Web sites external to NIOSH do not constitute NIOSH endorsement of the sponsoring organizations or their programs or products. Furthermore, NIOSH is not responsible for the content of these Web sites.

Ordering Information

To receive documents or other information about occupational safety and health topics, contact NIOSH at

Telephone: **1–800–CDC–INFO** (1–800–232–4636)
TTY: 1–888–232–6348
e-mail: cdcinfo@cdc.gov

or visit the NIOSH Web site at **www.cdc.gov/niosh**.

For a monthly update on news at NIOSH, subscribe to NIOSH *eNews* by visiting **www.cdc.gov/niosh/eNews**.

DHHS (NIOSH) Publication No. 2008–134

June 2008

SAFER • HEALTHIER • PEOPLE™

CONTENTS

Page

Executive summary 1

Background 3

Introduction 4

Permitting 5

    Structural design 5

    Impoundment location considerations 5

    Introductory information 6

    General permit information 7

    Geotechnical considerations 7

        Geology 8

        Competence of the strata 8

        Sensitivity to water 9

        Pillar stability 9

        Grouting of the strata surrounding the bulkhead 10

        Roof stability 11

        Removal of material affected by water 11

        Effects of mining near the bulkhead site 12

    Maps and drawings 12

    System design 13

        Safety factors 13

        Fluid pressure rating 14

        Ventilation seal regulations 15

        Seismic loading 16

        Impoundment perimeter 16

        Water sampling 17

    Bulkhead structure design 17

        Structural resistance 20

        Flexural design of reinforced concrete bulkheads 20

        Thick concrete bulkhead plugs 21

        Shear design of reinforced concrete bulkheads 22

    Cement selection 23

    Conduits passing through bulkhead structures 24

    Method to control fluid elevation 25

    Leakage prevention 26

    Emergency response plan 27

    Summary 30

Construction 30

    Site preparation 30

    Construction techniques 31

    Training 32

    Quality control plan 33

    Summary 34

CONTENTS—Continued

Page

Monitoring 34
    Routine inspections 35
    Head pressure 35
    Pump performance 36
    Drainage and monitoring pipes 36
    Leakage 37
    Deflection 37
    Summary 37
Conclusions 38
Acknowledgments 41
References 42
Appendix A.—Additional guidance for maps and drawings 45
Appendix B.—Sample bulkhead inspection sheet 48

ILLUSTRATIONS

1. Three basic designs used for bulkheads constructed in underground coal mines 17
2. Reinforced concrete "cap" bulkhead installed across drift opening to contain an unexpected
    inrush of water or slurry from surface impoundment above the abandoned mine works 18
3. Grouted rock bulkhead installed across drift opening 18

TABLES

1. Types of approved bulkhead designs used in U.S. underground coal mines 19
2. Types of approved materials used to construct bulkheads 19
3. Attack on concrete by soils and water containing various sulfate concentrations 24

ACRONYMS AND ABBREVIATIONS USED IN THIS REPORT

ACI	American Concrete Institute
ARMPS	Analysis of Retreat Mining Pillar Stability
ASTM	American Society for Testing and Materials
CMRR	Coal Mine Roof Rating
ISRM	International Society of Rock Mechanics
LVDT	linear variable displacement transducer
MSDS	material safety data sheet
MSHA	Mine Safety and Health Administration
NIOSH	National Institute for Occupational Safety and Health
OSM	Office of Surface Mining, Reclamation, and Enforcement
PPE	personal protective equipment
PVC	polyvinyl chloride

UNIT OF MEASURE ABBREVIATIONS USED IN THIS REPORT

ft	foot
gpm	gallon per minute
in	inch
in^2	square inch
in^2/ft^2	square inch per square foot
lb	pound
lb/ft^2	pound per square foot
lb/ft^3	pound per cubic foot
lb-in	pound-inch
ppm	parts per million
psi	pound-force per square inch

GUIDELINES FOR PERMITTING, CONSTRUCTION, AND MONITORING OF RETENTION BULKHEADS IN UNDERGROUND COAL MINES

By Samuel P. Harteis, P.E.,[1] Dennis R. Dolinar,[2] and Terence M. Taylor, P.E.[3]

EXECUTIVE SUMMARY

Many mining operations rely on retention bulkheads to provide a barrier between impounded water and active mine workings. However, bulkhead failures can cause catastrophic flooding that puts the underground workforce at risk. Underground observations and evaluations of existing bulkheads indicate that a systems approach is required when building an underground water or slurry retention system. In addition to engineering the bulkhead, the designer must ensure the quality control of materials and workmanship of the bulkhead, the reaction of the mine strata when exposed to water under pressure, and methods to monitor the performance of the retention system.

Researchers from the National Institute for Occupational Safety and Health (NIOSH), with the assistance of the Mine Safety and Health Administration (MSHA), conducted an extensive review of bulkhead permits submitted to the MSHA Technical Support office in Bruceton, PA. In addition, the researchers visited accessible bulkhead installations at underground mining operations to gather information related to construction practices, maintenance issues, and monitoring and emergency response procedures. Several key items were identified that must be considered when permitting the installation of an underground fluid retention system.

- In general, bulkheads are installed across mine openings to create an area for an underground impoundment. At many operations, the underground impoundment becomes a sealed area once the bulkheads are installed. Current MSHA ventilation regulations require seal structures to withstand pressures of 50 psi if the atmosphere behind the seal is monitored and maintained inert. If the atmosphere is not inert, the seal structure must withstand pressures up to 120 psi [72 Fed. Reg.[4] 28795 (2007)]. The calculations and design for these structures can be complex and should be completed by a registered professional engineer with a strong background in structural design and a working knowledge of underground mining operations.

---

[1]Research Engineer (Mining Engineer), Pittsburgh Research Laboratory, National Institute for Occupational Safety and Health, Pittsburgh, PA.

[2]Lead Research Engineer (Mining Engineer), Pittsburgh Research Laboratory, National Institute for Occupational Safety and Health, Pittsburgh, PA.

[3]Senior Civil Engineer, Mine Safety and Health Administration, Technical Support, Pittsburgh, PA.

[4]*Federal Register.* See Fed. Reg. in references.

- The underground impoundment should be located at an elevation that will still permit personnel to evacuate to the surface if a breach occurs. If the facility is to be used as a live fluid handling system, it must have adequate storage capacity to handle anticipated peak inflow rates, which includes fluid being directed into the impoundment from the operation and anticipated inflow of fluid from adjacent mine works and surface sources. The system should provide a minimum reserve capacity to allow for electrical interruptions, mechanical failures, and other conditions that prevent discharging fluid from the impoundment. The barrier pillars that form the perimeter of the impoundment must have the proper strength and geological qualities to remain stable for the life of the impoundment. Calculations and testing must be conducted to verify these strength and geological characteristics.

- The bulkhead design must consider all sources of fluid that could increase the pressure on the structure and design for the maximum anticipated fluid level. The selected bulkhead construction material must be compatible with the fluid impounded. To control leakage, contact pressure grouting of the bulkhead/strata interface is recommended for long-term installations, and all conduits that pass through the bulkhead must contain antiseep collars and be corrosion-resistant. If cementitious material is selected for bulkhead construction, steps must be taken to control the heat of hydration.

- Strata supporting the bulkheads must be tested and deemed competent to remain stable for the life of the impoundment. Roof, rib, and floor material that is affected by water, damaged, or fractured by mining must be removed from the mine floor beneath the bulkhead. Ring pressure grouting is recommended for all long-term installations to control leakage through the strata surrounding the bulkhead. Mining underlying seams in the vicinity of the impoundment should be minimized and conducted in such a manner that will not reduce the capability of the bulkheads to retain fluid. Standard precautions associated with mining under bodies of water must also be taken.

- A detailed construction plan that covers each phase of the construction process from site preparation through completion of the installation must be developed. This plan should include quality control procedures to ensure that the construction materials meet standards required by the design, the proper construction techniques are followed, the required procedures are followed for materials mixed on site, and the photographic and written documentation is obtained and recorded during construction of the installation.

- Routine monitoring the performance of the underground fluid retention system is essential and will be required for the life of the impoundment. Pressure transducers connected to monitoring systems that continuously record the static pressure exerted on the bulkhead are recommended. System designs should include provisions for monitoring inflow and discharge rates, pumping operations, and measurable leakage rates. For impoundments that cannot be monitored through underground workings, surface monitoring wells must be established to track fluid levels.

The guidelines in this report are to be used as a tool to identify areas or conditions that could impact the long-term stability of an underground fluid retention system and to give direction in addressing these situations. Although an attempt has been made to identify the common design considerations, it should not be considered an all-encompassing list. Each operation has unique features that could impact the integrity of an underground impoundment, and the responsibility of identifying these site-specific conditions rests with the permit applicant. The goal is to assist the permit applicant through the process of developing a complete permit package for a fluid retention system that is adequately designed for the operation and provides a safe environment for the workforce.

BACKGROUND

Underground mines install bulkheads across openings for a variety of purposes. Bulkheads are most commonly used as a dam to contain water or liquidlike mine wastes (tailings or slurry) in abandoned mine workings. Bulkheads are also used as regulators to restrict the flow of water from abandoned mine workings into active mining operations. In some cases where abandoned mine workings are located beneath a refuse impoundment, bulkheads are installed at the surface entrances to the abandoned mine workings. These structures are designed to prevent the outflow of water and liquidlike mine wastes from the openings if the overlying surface impoundment should break through into the abandoned mine workings. Failure of any of these bulkheads could result in a disastrous inundation, with the potential for significant loss of life or property and possible damage to the environment.

Although no mining fatalities have been directly attributable to bulkhead failures, recent catastrophic mine inundations have underscored the need for sound engineering practices in the design and maintenance of these structures to decrease the potential for loss of life. On March 1, 1991, bulkheads designed and constructed to impound water were installed across the main entries between the abandoned Raccoon No. 3 Mine and the downdip and active Meigs No. 31 Mine in Ohio. On July 11, 1993, an inundation occurred at the Meigs No. 31 Mine when these bulkheads failed. Fortunately, early discovery of the failure and a sufficiently slow waterflow enabled all miners to escape from the mine. A subsequent MSHA investigation [Tulanowski et al. 1993] indicated that the likely failure mechanism was erosion (or piping) along the concrete/fireclay interface at the base of the bulkhead.

In 2002, the U.S. Congress requested that the National Research Council investigate the October 11, 2000, failure of the Martin County Coal Corp. impoundment near Inez, KY. In this incident, over 250 million gallons of impounded slurry broke through strata into an abandoned area of an underground mine, then broke through a bulkhead, and ultimately discharged into nearby creeks and streams, causing significant environmental damage. Fortunately, the incident caused no injuries or fatalities. Wu et al. [2003] noted that several other breakthroughs of slurry into underground mine workings similar to this incident have occurred in recent years.

To understand the requirements for bulkhead installations and the permitting process, NIOSH researchers examined the bulkhead permits submitted to the MSHA Technical Support office in Bruceton, PA. Researchers then visited MSHA district offices and state mining agencies, and also contacted engineering consulting firms to document permitting information and to determine the number of bulkheads and their locations in the U.S. coalfields. A total of 35 bulkhead sites (existing or in the permit stage) were identified in the 11 MSHA districts.

Of the 35 identified bulkhead sites, 17 installations created an active water reservoir or controlled waterflow from abandoned mines, 6 facilitated surface refuse disposal facilities, 4 sealed off underground areas for slurry injection, and 3 created impoundments in an attempt to extinguish a mine fire. Permits were issued for three sites where bulkheads were not constructed. The remaining two sites were in the permitting stage [Harteis and Dolinar 2006].

Prior to construction of any bulkhead, MSHA and state mining agencies must review and approve the design. This usually entails submission of a proposed design by a registered professional engineer for evaluation by MSHA's Technical Support Group. Once the initial review is complete, the permit package is routinely returned to the operator with a request for additional information and clarifications. In many cases, the initial permit submission focuses on the bulkhead and contains limited information on the support systems.

This NIOSH Information Circular was developed for operations that need to construct an underground impoundment system, as well as for those that currently operate one. Much of the information contained in this report is geared toward the permitting aspect. However, information on monitoring and emergency response planning and training could be useful to operations that currently have underground impoundments.

In many instances, bulkheads serve the same purpose as ventilation seals until fluid builds up behind them. In most instances, the pressure requirements for a ventilation seal will exceed the pressure requirements for the bulkhead. When developing the permit, contact MSHA for the latest ventilation seal requirements and address the design requirements as they pertain to the proposed installation.

INTRODUCTION

NIOSH researchers, with assistance from MSHA, conducted an extensive review of bulkhead permits submitted to MSHA's Technical Support office in Bruceton, PA. The review indicated that once the need for an underground fluid retention structure was identified, considerable engineering hours were spent designing bulkheads that were capable of safely withstanding the pressure created from the estimated water head. Less effort was placed on addressing the surrounding strata's reaction to the impoundment, future mine plans, long-term ground control, monitoring systems, and emergency response. Upon completing a review of the bulkhead permits, accessible bulkheads at underground mining operations in Alabama, Indiana, Kentucky, Maryland, and West Virginia were visited to gather information on monitoring methods, Emergency Response Plans, and construction practices. Review of the permit packages combined with comments from mine operators, consulting engineers, and permit reviewers identified the need to develop guidelines for permitting, construction, and monitoring of retention bulkheads in underground coal mines.

This report is based on information obtained during research and field investigations and is designed to guide the mine operator or permit engineer through the process of designing and permitting an underground fluid retention system. Aside from assisting in bulkhead design, this report will give guidance in addressing geologic aspects, available monitoring devices, considerations for developing Emergency Response Plans, and other permitting issues. These guidelines are to be used as a tool to identify areas or conditions that could impact the long-term stability of the system and to give direction in addressing these situations. Although this report has identified many of the common design considerations for an underground impoundment system, it should not be considered an all-encompassing guideline. Each operation has unique features that could impact the integrity of an underground impoundment, and the responsibility of identifying these site-specific conditions rests with the permit applicant. These bulkhead guidelines are divided into three main topic areas: (1) permitting, (2) construction, and (3) monitoring.

PERMITTING

Structural Design

Of the 30 sites where bulkheads were installed, 16 were designed to withstand head pressures less than 25 psi, 7 were designed to withstand pressures greater than 25 psi but less than 50 psi, 5 were designed to withstand pressures greater than 50 psi but less than 120 psi, and 2 were designed to withstand pressures greater than 120 psi. At many of the operations, bulkheads seal off abandoned mine works. Prior to the 2006 Sago Mine explosion in West Virginia, ventilation seals were required to withstand an explosion overpressure of 20 psi. Although some of the bulkheads were designed to withstand head pressures less than 20 psi with adequate safety factors, their basic designs were capable of withstanding a 20-psi explosion over-pressure. Current MSHA ventilation regulations require seal structures to withstand pressures from 50 psi if the atmosphere behind the bulkhead is monitored and maintained inert. If the atmosphere is not monitored and not maintained inert, the seal structure must withstand pressures up to 120 psi [72 Fed. Reg. 28795 (2007)].

A review of the existing bulkhead designs indicates that a variety of material and construction techniques have been used in the past. They range from low-strength monolithic concrete plugs to high-strength reinforced concrete slabs and include composite designs with masonry wall forms that use limestone and polyurethane for the core material. Some designs were very basic and required minimal engineering, while others required expertise in structural design. Designs of bulkheads that meet or exceed MSHA ventilation regulations require the expertise of a registered professional engineer with a background in structural design and a working knowledge of underground mining operations. If these skills are not available in-house, retain the services of a consulting engineer with experience in performing work of this type.

> **Bulkhead design and related calculations must be performed by a registered professional engineer with a strong background in structural design and a working knowledge of underground mining operations.**

Impoundment Location Considerations

At most operations, the physical location of the underground impoundment and bulkheads will be limited by the existing mine works. Key factors to consider before finalizing the impoundment location are:

- The impoundment elevation must be such that if a breach occurs, the fluid escaping the impoundment will not trap miners and prevent their escape to the surface. Impoundment locations that place active mine works and employees in the path of fluid escaping the impoundment should be avoided.

- Routine monitoring of the bulkhead is required for the life of the system. Determine the route that inspectors will travel to conduct routine inspections of the fluid retention system, and perform a visual examination of the roof, floor, ribs, and existing ground control measures in these areas. Note conditions that would restrict access to the bulkhead. Avoid areas that cannot be made safe for routine travel.

- The impoundment must be of sufficient capacity to adequately store or handle the peak volume of fluid anticipated during normal operations, with additional storage for unexpected events. It is recommended that the system maintain a reserve capacity to provide storage for periods when fluid cannot be removed. The reserve capacity should be of sufficient size to provide time for repair or replacement of system components, power outages, and performance of routine maintenance. If the system design is such that major components could be out of service for extended periods, the operation must make provision to obtain critical spare parts on short notice or increase the reserve capacity accordingly.

- Electricity may be required to power monitoring devices on the bulkhead and to operate pumps controlling the fluid level in the impoundment. Consider the cost and placement of electrical power at that location.

- The physical location of the bulkhead should be a minimum of 10 ft from the outby pillar corner.

> **The impoundment must be located at an elevation that will not trap miners and prevent their escape to the surface if a breach occurs. The fluid retention system should have a built-in reserve capacity to allow for periods when fluid cannot be removed.**

Introductory Information

The permit application will likely be reviewed by personnel who do not have firsthand knowledge of the operation. The introductory section will assist the permit reviewer in gaining knowledge of the mining operation and the proposed underground impoundment. The section consists of:

- A general information sheet that lists specific information for the operation such as the mine name, location, and associated ID and other permit numbers.

- An impoundment information sheet that summarizes key information related to the underground fluid retention system.

- A written overview that briefly discusses the need for the system, material to be impounded, source of the material, primary method of monitoring the system, plan to control fluid elevation, location of discharge point, and receiving stream or body of water, if applicable.

General Permit Information

Once the location is selected, the following detailed information must be included in the permit package. Include references to maps or drawings in the submission where necessary.

- A written discussion of the proposed impoundment location and how the elevation of the proposed impoundment relates to current and future mining activities should be provided. Include in the discussion actual mine floor elevations of the proposed impoundment area, bulkhead site elevations, and the maximum expected pool elevations.

- Using mine floor elevations, determine the route by which fluid will flow if the bulkhead system fails. Identify inundation areas where fluid will pool and areas that will potentially hinder evacuation of personnel through existing escapeways. The fluid flow path and pool areas should be indicated on the contour mine map that is detailed in Appendix A. If areas exist that have the potential to flood and block evacuation of personnel, designate alternate escapeways on this map and discuss other means available for personnel to escape to the surface or a safe location. This information should also be included in the Emergency Response section of the permit application.

- A written description of elevations of adjacent mine works and the proximity to the proposed impoundment should be provided. Include an evaluation of the possibility of fluid flowing into the impoundment area from adjacent mine works or from the impoundment into adjacent mine works. Discuss areas where retreat or longwall mining has occurred and open fractures may exist that will allow fluid transfer. Identify areas where barrier pillars that are less than 200 ft wide separate the impoundment from existing or projected mine works within the same seam. When writing this section, consider adjacent works that are within the same mining horizon, above and below. Keep in mind that fluid flow could occur through both the roof and floor strata that separate the seams. Also consider the possible effects of subsidence in underlying seams on the bulkheads.

Identify all mine works, both active and inactive, that could impact the amount of fluid flowing into and out of the proposed underground impoundment.

Geotechnical Considerations

Geotechnical information on site-specific conditions is required. It should be noted that some bulkheads have failed through the surrounding strata or along the strata/bulkhead interface. Therefore, an evaluation of the site geology, hydrology, and ground control issues will have to be conducted. Essentially, geotechnical data must be provided that demonstrate that the bulkhead is being placed in competent rock at a site that is stable and will remain stable for the life of the impoundment. Further, it must be shown that the site or the rock surrounding the bulkhead will not deteriorate because of the water or slurry retained behind the bulkhead or that there will not be excessive leakage through the strata or along the strata/bulkhead interface. Measures must be taken to minimize the effects of the impounded fluid on the rock, excessive leakage through the rock or bulkhead, or failure of the strata. A person who is competent and knowledgeable in the subject must conduct a thorough geotechnical site assessment.

Geology

Information on the site geology needs to be provided detailing the strata in the vicinity of the bulkhead. This includes a geologic log and description of the rock units in the immediate roof and floor and the thicknesses of those units. These geologic descriptions must be given to a depth at least to and through competent rock that is minimally affected by water. Competent rock must have sufficient strength to withstand the footprint of the bulkhead. In addition, the rock must not be fractured or degraded by the mining process, and the rock should not deteriorate significantly when exposed to the fluid retained by the bulkhead. Greater depths for the geologic description may be necessary depending on the potential depth of fluid penetration. Essentially, if there is a potential for a rock unit to be affected by the fluid retained in the impoundment, a description of that unit should be given. Conditions in the mined coal seam must also be described, including any partings in the seam and the cleat pattern that could affect the degree of leakage around the bulkhead.

Competence of the Strata

Physical property tests should be conducted on the roof and floor rock that show the strength of the different geologic units. Uniaxial compressive strength and point load index tests can be used [Rusnak and Mark 2000; ISRM 1985; ASTM 2004b]. The results of these tests will demonstrate the relative (between rock units) and general competence of the rock units. These tests should be conducted from material obtained in the vicinity of the site. If there is a potential for a shear failure along the bulkhead/strata interface or through the strata as a result of weak strata, shear strengths of the planes of weakness or weak layers need to be determined.

Floor failure and the resultant floor heave and convergence, if excessive, could have a detrimental impact on a bulkhead. Therefore, an analysis of the bearing capacity of the floor may need to be conducted. There are specific tests that can be used to determine the bearing capacity, or the ultimate bearing capacity can be estimated for clays from the moisture content [Su et al. 1993; Barney and Nair 1970; Speck 1981; Pytel 1994]. The bearing capacity can also be estimated from the cohesion and angle of internal friction of the material. A safety factor greater than 2 should be used in evaluating the potential for a bearing-capacity failure as recommended by Bieniawski [1992a] because of assumptions made about pillar load distribution. The effects of water on the strength of the floor material must also be considered.

> **Demonstrate that the bulkhead is being placed in competent rock at a site that will remain stable for the life of the impoundment. A trained professional with experience in performing this type of site assessment must conduct the evaluation.**

Sensitivity to Water

Often, the immediate floor or roof may consist of a fireclay, underclay, or mudstone that could be affected by water. Piping of water through a fireclay or along the bulkhead/fireclay interface was the most likely mechanism for the failure of one bulkhead that led to the flooding of a mine [Tulanowski et al. 1993].

Rocks that are directly in contact with the bulkhead or could affect the bulkhead performance as a result of the impounded fluid need to be tested to determine how sensitive the rocks are to the fluid. There are a number of tests that can be conducted to determine the effects of water on the rock. These include the slake durability test, weatherability test, Coal Mine Roof Rating (CMRR) immersion test, and clay dispersion test [Mark et al. 2002; Mark and Molinda 2007; Molinda et al. 2006; Harteis and Dolinar 2006; Unrug 1997; Sherard and Decker 1977; ASTM 2004a]. From the test results, it should be clearly stated to what degree the rock was affected by water and the impact on the bulkhead design. Essentially, the acceptable limits for the specific type of tests should be provided to explain if water would affect the rock and the bulkhead's ability to impound the water or slurry.

For the strata directly in contact with the bulkhead, the slake durability index should be in the medium-high or above categories (>85), and the CMRR immersion test results should be in the slightly to not-sensitive categories. However, it might not always be possible to locate the foot of the bulkhead in strata that are in these ranges. In that case, strata should be selected that are relatively less affected by water than the surrounding strata, or the degradable strata should be removed beneath the structures. Weatherability tests have shown that the types of strata that are most sensitive to water are generally the fireclays and the sandy shales [Molinda et al. 2006].

> **Strata directly in contact with the bulkhead should have a slake durability index of at least medium-high, and the CMRR should be in the slightly to not-sensitive categories.**

Pillar Stability

Coal pillars to which the bulkheads are anchored must remain stable for the life of the impoundment. Engineering calculations that demonstrate a sufficient safety factor for long-term stability of these pillars should be included. Computer software such as Analysis of Retreat Mining Pillar Stability (ARMPS) can be used to calculate a stability factor for the pillars for a regular mine pattern or layout [Mark and Chase 1997; NIOSH 2008a]. For more irregular mine layouts, the boundary-element program called LaModel can be used to calculate the pillar stresses and then, in combination with ARMPS, a stability or safety factor can be determined [Heasley and Chekan 1999; Heasley and Agioutantis 2007; NIOSH 2008b]. With ARMPS, the stability factor is the calculated pillar load divided by the calculated pillar strength. However, for ARMPS the suggested stability factors for successful mining apply only when a panel is retreat-mined and, therefore, are not relevant to pillars with bulkheads. Bieniawski [1992b] suggests using a stability factor of 2.0 for pillars in mains. Since these pillars in the mains are long-term stable structures, a minimum stability factor of 2.0 for the pillars surrounding the bulkhead seems to be appropriate. In general, most bulkheads have been installed only where development mining exists and the installations were sufficiently removed from more extensive mining so as to not see additional loads. Typically, extraction ratios vary from 0.33 to 0.55, with the ARMPS stability factor for the pillar systems ranging from 2.4 to 9.5 depending on the depth of the site.[5] These stability factors are based on dry conditions with no degradation of the floor, roof, or pillar strengths as a result of water. However, no known failures of pillars that contained bulkheads have occurred based on a recent survey of installed bulkheads in U.S. coal mines [Harteis and Dolinar 2006].

There is at least one case of pillar failure in a room-and-pillar panel where coal slurry was being injected [Ross et al. 1998].[6] The failure was attributed to the pillars punching into underclay in the floor, which was saturated with water. The underclay was approximately 3 ft thick and underlain by 7 ft of claystone. The initial dry-condition ARMPS stability factor was 2.3. Based on the analysis, the ARMPS stability factor was reduced to 1.09 when the pillar strength was degraded and the pillar height was increased as a result of the effects of the water on the underclay.

If underclay, fireclay, or other material exists in the floor or roof directly above or below the coal seam that is affected by water, the reaction to water of the roof or floor material on the pillar strength should be evaluated. This especially applies to room-and-pillar panels that are used for the impoundment. Additionally, the impacts of a resulting pillar failure (such as subsidence), the possible increased loads on the pillars containing the bulkheads, and the strata damage near bulkheads may have to be evaluated.

To assist in evaluating the potential for floor failure or floor heave, the bearing capacity of the floor must be determined. To reduce the potential for a bearing-capacity failure of the floor from the pillars, Bieniawski [1992a] suggests that safety factors should be greater than 2 because of assumptions made about the load distribution. These calculations must take into account any deterioration in the strength of the floor from the water.

> **Conduct and provide engineering calculations demonstrating that the coal pillars to which the bulkheads are anchored have a sufficient safety factor for long-term stability.**

Grouting of the Strata Surrounding the Bulkhead

Invariably there will be leakage of fluid through the surrounding strata. The amount of leakage depends on the geologic and strata conditions, the thickness of the bulkhead, and the water head. Ring grouting of the rock mass and coal seam will reduce the permeability of the strata and increase the length of the flow path for the fluid around the bulkhead. Due to the strata conditions and the potential for excessive leakage through the strata, grouting of the strata was done at 17 of the 30 bulkhead sites. However, of the 13 sites with no grouting of the strata, 3 of the bulkhead systems were installed in an emergency situation to flood the mines to put out a fire. At three other sites, the bulkheads were built as a secondary defense in case a surface

---

[5]The few bulkheads installed in barrier pillars, along with those near or at the seam outcrops, were not included in this ARMPS analysis.

[6]The panel had been sealed, but bulkheads to retain slurry were not installed. When the pillars failed, the panel collapsed and slurry breached the seals.

impoundment would break through into the underground workings. Under normal conditions, water or slurry is not retained behind these bulkheads. Two sites constructed bulkheads in abandoned mine openings to extend the life of coarse refuse disposal facilities. During normal operations, neither site impounds fluid. Finally at one site with no grouting, the strata under the bulkheads failed most likely because of piping and resulted in flooding of the mine. Therefore, based on current and prudent engineering practice, ring grouting of the strata around the bulkhead is recommended for all bulkheads designed for long-term impoundments of water and slurry.

Grouting is usually done through small-diameter boreholes drilled into the roof, coal, and floor in a ring pattern around the perimeter of the bulkhead. The depth of the grouting will depend on the strata and fluid head, but will typically be 6–30 ft. Sufficient holes should be drilled around the opening to establish an adequate grout curtain that minimizes leakage.

> **Ring grouting should be conducted for all long-term underground impoundments.**

Roof Stability

Additional roof support must be installed on both the wet and dry sides of the bulkhead. On the wet side, there is an increased potential for roof falls if the roof rock is affected by water. A roof fall would expose additional roof above the bulkhead to the water and possibly form a pathway around the bulkhead. On the dry side, additional support must be installed to provide safe passage for personnel, increase the long-term stability of the strata, and reduce the potential of a roof fall that could extend laterally over the bulkhead. Additional roof support can be in the form of standing supports, roof bolts, longer roof bolts, or cable bolts and a combination of these roof control measures should be evaluated. If standing support is used, the stability of the roof and floor under the support must be considered.

> **Provide additional roof support on both sides of the bulkheads to increase the long-term stability of the strata.**

Removal of Material Affected by Water

If the immediate roof or floor is affected by water or fractured and damaged by mining, the material should be removed from the footprint of the bulkhead. This is especially true for floor material where fireclays and underclays often exist that can be severely damaged by mining and can be degraded from exposure to water or slurry. Further, the design of the bulkhead may require hitching into the surrounding rock mass. In any case, the material must be removed to a depth where the bulkhead will be in contact with and keyed into competent rock that is not or is only minimally affected by water. For the installations reviewed by NIOSH, the depth of material removed from the floor either for placing the bulkhead on competent strata or for hitching the bulkhead into the surrounding strata ranged from 6 in to 4 ft. Loose rib material should also be removed to allow the bulkhead to be in contact with a solid coal rib. Trenching into the ribs may also be done to allow the bulkhead to be installed against more competent coal. At one site visited by researchers, the coal ribs were very soft and did not permit trenching. However, the operation chose to stabilize the ribs by polyurethane grouting the coal seam from the bulkhead to the outby rib corner and through the first outby crosscut.

On the dry side of the bulkhead, the floor may be trenched along the pillar to the same depth as the material removed from under the bulkhead. The trench is then filled with concrete to a height that is several inches above the pillar/floor interface. This additional height prevents or minimizes leakage along the floor/pillar interface. The concrete fill in the floor trench should be doweled into the floor strata to resist seepage uplift forces. This trench can reduce the potential for leakage and piping under the pillar near the bulkhead. At one U.S. mine, trenches were installed for a distance of up to 9 ft from the outby side of the bulkhead. This resulted in an overall path length of 15 ft for the fluid, which included the thickness of the bulkhead. Although this technique is not common, it can be effective in increasing the seepage resistance as long as the excavation method does not adversely impact the strength of the adjacent strata.

> **Remove immediate roof or floor material from the footprint of the bulkhead that is affected by water or damaged and fractured by mining.**

Effects of Mining Near the Bulkhead Site

The effects of any subsequent mining in the same or adjacent seams near the bulkhead must be evaluated. Since any resulting strata movement or loads need to be kept to a minimum, additional nearby mining must be limited [Kirkwood and Wu 1995] and avoided, if possible. The influence of any overlying or underlying mine workings must also be analyzed. Particular attention must be given to any underlying mine workings, because any collapse or subsidence from these underlying works could cause significant strata movement in the overlying seam [Kendorski 1993, 2006; Mark 2007]. Therefore, prudent engineering practice requires that underlying works in the vicinity of the bulkheads or impoundment be very limited or non-existent. Any mining conducted in underlying seams in the vicinity of the fluid retention system must not reduce the capability of the bulkheads to retain fluid, and precautions associated with mining under bodies of water must be taken.

> **To maintain the integrity of the strata supporting the underground fluid retention system, any mining conducted in the vicinity of the bulkheads and the impounded fluid in underlying seams should be very limited.**

Maps and Drawings

Various maps and drawings will be required for the permit package. This includes a map of the workings adjacent to the impoundment location, maps of mine works located above and below the proposed impoundment, and surface overlay maps. Keep in mind that the permit reviewer may not have firsthand knowledge of the mine or operation and will require clarifications to information provided on the maps that is unclear or illegible. Additional guidance for maps and drawings is included in Appendix A.

System Design

When developing the design and list of components required for the fluid retention system, the engineer is required to select materials and designs that perform their intended task with a reasonable margin of safety that will account for variations in materials and any unseen conditions. Although general guidance is provided in this report, the engineers must make selections based on knowledge of the geologic setting for the system, future mining plans, past experience with materials, recommendations from the manufacturers, and sound engineering practices that provide the operation with a safe and efficient system.

Safety Factors

Minimum design safety factors should be based on using construction materials and analytical techniques with a known history of performance, such as cement-based materials. Reinforced concrete structures should be designed in accordance with the most recent versions of the American Concrete Institute's (ACI) Code 318 and 350 [ACI 2005, 2006]. ACI 318 is the general building code for structural concrete, and ACI 350 is the code for environmental structures. The codes are based on the ultimate strength design concept in which load factors are applied to the loads and strength reduction factors (Φ) are applied to the strength to account for the uncertainty in predicting the material strength and the resistance or capacity of the structure. For example, when the fluid has a maximum controllable level, the hydrostatic loading should be multiplied by a minimum load factor of 1.4. The strength reduction factors vary depending on the type of strength under consideration. For example, when evaluating the shear strength of the structure, $\Phi = 0.75$; when checking the flexural strength, $\Phi = 0.9$. For nonreinforced concrete plug-type bulkheads, load factors and strength reduction factors are generally not applied. Rather, an overall safety factor is applied so that the resistance of the structure is at least two times the force from the external loading. The material strength should be based on a lower bound value. Documentation of material properties and material testing results should be included in the permit package to substantiate the values used in the structural calculations.

> **Reinforced concrete structures should be designed in accordance with the most recent versions of ACI 318 and 350.**
>
> **Nonreinforced concrete structures should be designed so that the resistance of the structure is at least two times the force from the external loading.**

13

Fluid Pressure Rating

The amount of fluid pressure that a bulkhead must resist is equal to the static pressure applied by the column of fluid being restrained by the structure. To estimate this value, determine the maximum elevation that the fluid could reach within the impoundment. Next, determine the elevation of the mine floor where the bulkhead(s) will be constructed. Subtract the mine floor elevation at the lowest bulkhead from the maximum fluid elevation to determine the maximum head pressure applied to the bulkhead. The following equation can be used to calculate the maximum pressure on the bulkhead:

$$P_{mw} = D_f H_w \tag{1}$$

where P_{mw} = maximum fluid pressure, lb/ft^2,
D_f = density of fluid, lb/ft^3,
and H_w = height of water, ft.

If the fluid is a mixture of solids and liquids, tests should be conducted to determine the density of the slurry and this value should be used as the value for D_f. When the fluid is water, the density is 62.4 lb/ft^3, and for a 40-ft head the maximum pressure on the bulkhead would be 2,496 lb/ft^2. To convert this pressure to pounds per square inch, the value is divided by 144 in^2/ft^2. The resulting pressure is 17.3 psi.

The average pressure on the lowest bulkhead in a set can be calculated from the following equation:

$$P_{aw} = D_f (H_w - \tfrac{1}{2} H_b) \tag{2}$$

where P_{aw} = average fluid pressure, lb/ft^2,
and H_b = height of bulkhead, ft.

In the above example, for an 8-ft-high bulkhead the average pressure on the bulkhead would be 2,246 lb/ft^2 (15.6 psi). However, it is recommended that the maximum pressure be used for design.

When determining the maximum fluid elevation, consider exterior sources of water or fluid that could enter the impoundment area through the coal seam or surrounding strata. Some common sources to consider are:

- Impounded water in adjacent mines
- Surface bodies of water, such as ponds, lakes, impoundments, or bodies of water
- Flowing water sources, such as creeks, streams, and rivers
- Natural aquifers

One of the operations visited by NIOSH was conducting room-and-pillar mining in a seam that was underlain by abandoned mine works. Although the seams were separated by 100 ft of strata, the elevation of the lower mine portal was higher than the elevation of the upper-seam mine portal. When pumping ceased in the lower seam, the water elevation rose to a point where water from the lower seam flowed into the upper seam through fractures in the strata created by longwall mining in the lower seam. In this case, the bulkhead must be designed to withstand the pressure of impounded water in the seam plus any additional pressure that could be applied from water in the lower seam. Breakthrough potential bulkheads are bulkheads designed to regulate the flow of water or slurry in the event that a surface impoundment breaks through into underground mine works. They have to withstand the force that could be applied from the fluid in the surface impoundment at its maximum elevation.

With these calculations, include a discussion of surface and subsurface sources of fluid that could impact the underground fluid retention system. Detail any fluid sources that have the potential to increase the static head on the bulkhead(s), and include the resulting additional static head in the calculations. If surface or subsurface sources of fluid exist but do not have the potential to impact the underground impoundment, state the reasons or logic that led to this conclusion. Give specific information such as the length or distance of interburden between the seam and body of water, type of strata, and other geologic information. Keep in mind that areas where retreat or longwall mining has occurred have great potential to transfer fluid from one seam to another.

> **The maximum fluid elevation must include consideration for exterior sources of water or fluid that could enter the impoundment area through the coal seam or surrounding strata.**

Ventilation Seal Regulations

Bulkheads installed across mine entries may seal off abandoned mine works. Current MSHA regulations require ventilation seals to withstand pressures of 50 psi if the atmosphere behind the seals is monitored and maintained inert. Seals designed to 120 psi are required if the atmosphere is not monitored and not maintained inert [72 Fed. Reg. 28795 (2007)]. Gas sampling pipes for monitoring the atmosphere within the sealed area may also be required until the fluid level exceeds the elevation of the sample or monitoring pipe. The permit applicant must research both state and federal regulations related to sealing abandoned mine workings and institute these requirements in the design of the bulkheads. Although these structures may be designed to withstand explosive forces from 50 to 120 psi, it should not be construed to mean that they will resist the same static forces applied by long-term fluid loading. Compared to ventilation seals, bulkhead designs need to address additional concerns, such as how seepage through the roof, floor, and ribs and constant fluid pressure may affect the strength of the anchorage. Failure of roof, floor, and ribs due to water pressure, hydraulic fracturing, and internal erosion are examples of failure mechanisms that must be considered for bulkheads.

> **Bulkheads that also function as mine ventilation seals may be required to meet the federal regulations covering these structures.**

Seismic Loading

When a bulkhead is located in a seismically active area, seismic loads need to be considered. The bulkhead design should consider both inertial and hydrodynamic forces that result from an earthquake. Inertial forces are related to the increase in static pressure caused by accelerating the bulkhead. Hydrodynamic forces are related to the increase in static pressure caused by accelerating the water mass behind the bulkhead. Both of these should be added to the static head pressure exerted on the bulkhead by the impounded fluid. Additional information can be found in the *Standard Handbook for Civil Engineers* [Merritt et al. 1996].

Impoundment Perimeter

In the earlier "Fluid Pressure Rating" section, the hydrostatic head generated by the fluid in the impoundment was calculated. The main reason for calculating this value is to properly design the bulkheads. However, the majority of the impoundment perimeter will normally consist of coal in the form of barrier pillars. In the permit package, include calculations confirming that the barrier is of sufficient width to support the roof and maintain the separation between the impoundment and other workings, either existing or projected.

A guideline developed and used successfully by U.K. coal operators [King and Whittaker 1971] is that the width of the barrier pillar should be one-tenth of the overburden plus 45 ft:

$$W_p = \frac{h}{10} + 45 \tag{3}$$

where W_p = width of the barrier pillar, ft,
and h = depth in feet below the surface [Peng 1986].

The Ashley, or Mine Inspector, Formula was established by a seven-member commission for the Commonwealth of Pennsylvania. The main objective of the commission was to develop a method of designing coal barriers to impound water and protect active mines from unexpected inundations. From the findings of the commission, the minimum width of the barrier pillar is expressed as:

$$W_p = 20 + 4T + 0.1D \tag{4}$$

where T = average thickness of the coal seam, ft,
and D = depth of overburden or the height of water head, ft [Chekan 1985].

> **In the permit package, include calculations confirming that the barrier pillar is of sufficient width to support the roof and maintain the separation between the impoundment and other workings, either existing or projected.**

16

Water Sampling

A chemical analysis of the water to be impounded (pH, alkalinity, total suspended solids, and specific conductance) must be completed by a certified lab and the results included in the permit package. If it is likely that other sources of water will be entering the impoundment from adjacent mines or surface water features, obtain current chemical analysis from these sources. A copy of the analysis is required to verify that bulkhead material selection is compatible with the fluid impounded.

Bulkhead Structure Design

The primary bulkhead designs for underground use are tapered plugs, parallel plugs, notched slabs (Figure 1), or variations of these basic designs [Garrett and Campbell Pitt 1958]. When bulkheads are installed at mine entrances on the surface to control fluid, other types are considered. One option is to construct a reinforced concrete structure near or in front of the opening to "cap" off the opening (Figure 2) [Harteis and Dolinar 2006]. A second option is to pneumatically stow crushed limestone in the entry between two concrete block walls and inject grout or polyurethane into the crushed limestone to form a watertight design (Figure 3) [Harteis and Dolinar 2006].

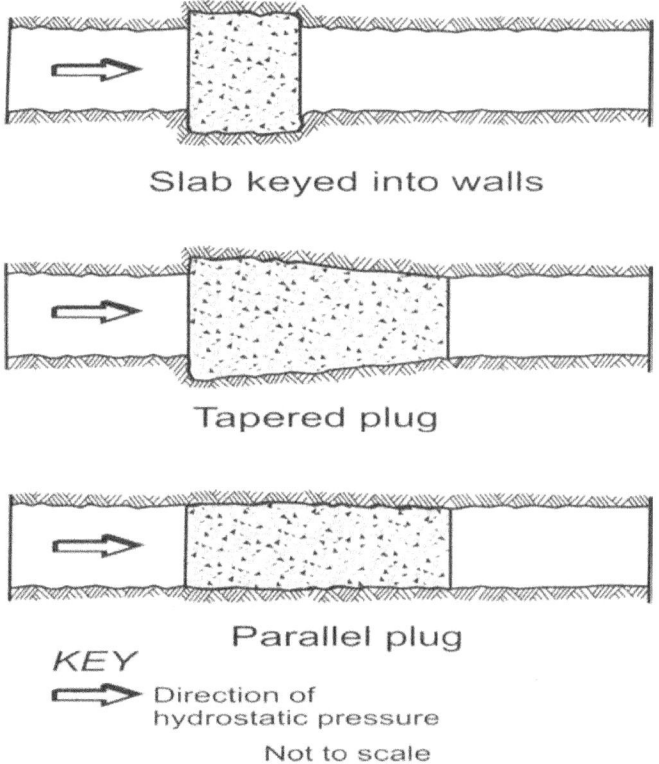

Figure 1.—Three basic designs used for bulkheads constructed in underground coal mines.

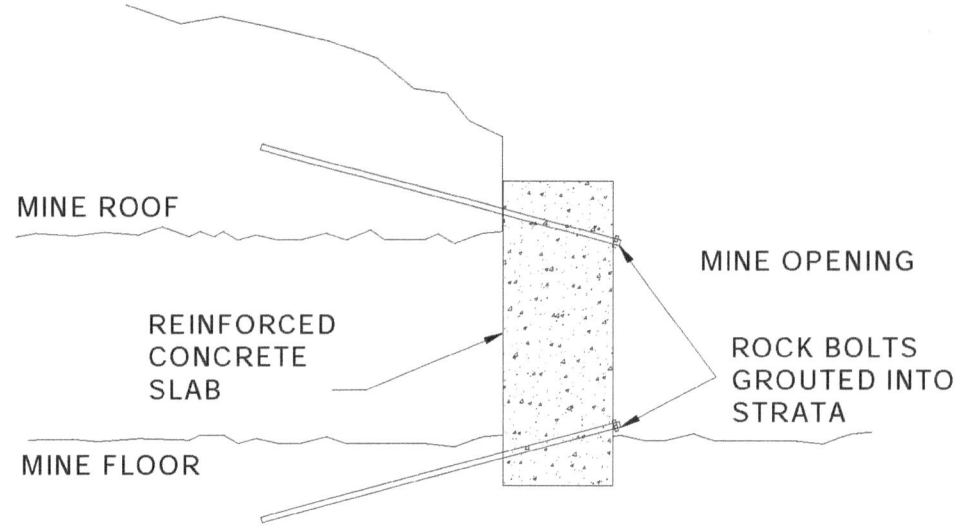

Figure 2.—Reinforced concrete "cap" bulkhead installed across drift opening to contain an unexpected inrush of water or slurry from surface impoundment above the abandoned mine works.

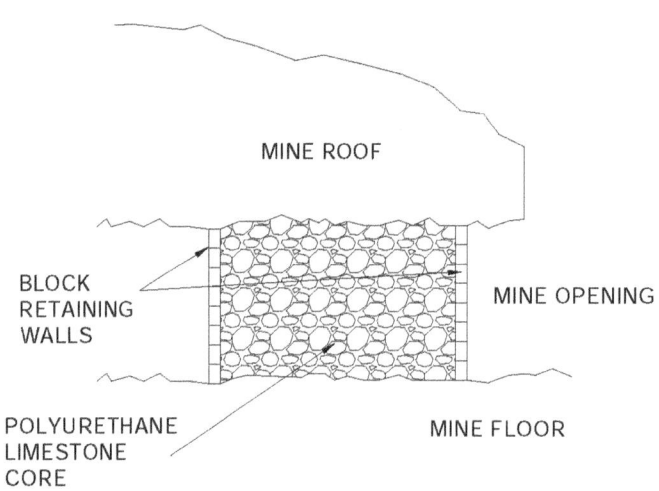

Figure 3.—Grouted rock bulkhead installed across drift opening.

The design that best suits the site-specific application depends on several variables. These include the anticipated water or slurry load (head pressure); explosion loading, if required; accessibility to the site from underground as well as from the surface; rib, roof, and floor conditions; floor heave; convergence; material handling restraints; and cost. Table 1 gives a breakdown of the bulkhead designs currently in use at U.S. mine sites.

Table 1.—Types of approved bulkhead designs used in U.S. underground coal mines

MSHA district	No. of bulkhead sites	Parallel plug	Tapered plug	Notched slab	Grouted rock	Cap
1	0					
2	7	1		6		
3	4	3		1		
4	6		2	2	1	1
5	3			3		
6	3	1		1		1
7	0					
8	1			1		
9	1		1			
10	4	1		3		
11	4	2		2		
TOTAL	33	8	3	19	1	2

A range of building materials have been used in bulkhead construction (see Table 2). Material selection depends on the bulkhead design selected, accessibility to the installation site, and cost.

Table 2.—Types of approved materials used to construct bulkheads

MSHA district	Concrete	Cementitious foam	Poly-urethane limestone	Poly-urethane	Masonry	Shotcrete
1						
2	4		1	1	1	
3	2		1	1		
4	2	2	1			1
5	1		2			
6	2		1			
7						
8			1			
9	1					
10	1		3			
11	2	1	1			
TOTAL	15	3	11	2	1	1

Structural Resistance

Considering the types of loading, the bulkhead must be designed to have the structural capacity to resist the forces acting on it with a safety factor consistent with the degree of uncertainty and the consequences of failure. The bulkhead must be able to resist the shear and bending stress caused by the pressure acting on the face of the bulkhead. The bending stress in both directions (roof-to-floor and rib-to-rib) can be calculated based on the edge restraints of a plate or slab and the relative dimensions of width and length [Timoshenko and Woinowsky-Kreiger 1959; Young 1989]. For thick members relative to span, Young [1989] provides guidance on stress multipliers for deep members. In addition to resisting the lateral loads, the bulkhead should have the capacity to resist the vertical bearing loads caused by mine roof convergence and stress transfer.

For thin bulkheads installed in typical openings with a cross-sectional width at least two times greater than the height of the opening, with adequate edge connections provided at the mine roof and floor, the bulkheads can be designed as a one-way slab spanning between the roof and floor. For aspect ratios of entry width to height less than 2, the bulkhead can be designed for two-way behavior provided there is also adequate anchorage to the rib strata. Reinforcement to account for temperature and shrinkage stresses would still be necessary in the rib-to-rib direction if one-way behavior is designed in the roof-to-floor direction. Regardless of the width-to-height ratio, diagonal reinforcement steel should be placed in the bulkhead corners to control cracking from twisting moments. Further, designers are cautioned that despite the load path direction assumed, if the mine roof, floor, and ribs are properly notched, or if the steel bar reinforcing mats near the inby and outby faces are adequately doweled into the surrounding strata, then it is possible to develop negative moment bending stresses at the edges of the restrained bulkhead slab. The negative steel (i.e., the steel bars near the inby "wet side" face) should be sized to resist negative moment bending stresses.

Reinforced concrete structures should be designed in accordance with the most recent versions of ACI 318 and 350. The codes are based on ultimate strength design, which entails applying uncertainty factors to the loads and strength reduction factors to the capacity of the structure. The design strength of the member must be greater than the required strength to ensure a safe design. For fluid pressure, the load factor is 1.4 when the maximum height of the water or slurry is controlled or conservatively estimated.

Flexural Design of Reinforced Concrete Bulkheads

The flexural design strength of a conventional/standard reinforced concrete member is given by the following expression:

$$M_d = \Phi A_s f_y \left(d - \frac{a}{2} \right) \tag{5}$$

where

M_d = flexural design strength, lb-in,

Φ = 0.9 (strength reduction factor),

A_s = area of tension reinforcement (in^2) per unit foot,

f_y = yield strength of the reinforcing steel, psi,

d = distance from extreme compression fiber to centroid of tension reinforcement, in,

and

a = depth of rectangular stress block at failure, in.

$$a = \frac{A_s f_y}{0.85 \ f_c' \ b} \tag{6}$$

where f'_c = specified compressive strength of concrete, psi,
and b = width of compression face of member (normally taken as 12 in for slabs), in.

For thicker bulkheads, the above capacity should be modified to reflect deep flexural member behavior. Thicker members have low span-to-thickness ratios, so the simple theory of linear stress distribution is no longer valid. According to Park and Paulay [1975], for simply supported members with span-to-depth (thickness) ratios less than or equal to 2, the internal lever arm can be calculated as:

$$z = 0.2(l + 2h) \qquad \text{when} \qquad 1 \le \frac{1}{h} \le 2 \tag{7}$$

$$z = 0.6 \ l \qquad \text{when} \qquad \frac{1}{h} \le 1 \tag{8}$$

where l = span distance centerline-to-centerline of two bearing points or 1.15 times the clear span (whichever is smaller), in,
  = h thickness of the bulkhead, in,
and z = internal lever arm, in.
Applying the revised lever arm value to the above standard flexural equation, the capacity can be estimated as:

$$M_d = \Phi A_s f_y z \tag{9}$$

The value of z should not be taken as greater than $[d - (a/2)]$. In addition, if the designer ensures that the end supports are fixed rather than simply supported, z values should be further adjusted [Park and Paulay 1975]. Winter and Nilson [1979] recommend that tension steel in a deep flexural member should be distributed over the bottom third of the member depth.

Thick Concrete Bulkhead Plugs

The shear resistance may be governed by the strength of the seal, the strength of the surrounding strata, or the contact interface between the two. In cases where there is no notching, the interface resistance may be governed by adhesion or friction. The South African plug formulas, which are based on the shear strength and bearing capacity of the bulkhead material and surrounding strata, are often used to evaluate the required length of thick bulkheads [Garrett and Campbell Pitt 1961]:

$$l = \frac{pab}{2(a+b)f_s} \tag{10}$$

$$l = \frac{pab}{(a+b)f_c} \tag{11}$$

where l = length of the bulkhead, ft,
                  p = hydraulic pressure on the bulkhead, psi,
                  a = width of the entry, ft,
                  b = height of the entry, ft,
                  f_s = minimum allowable shear strength of the strata or concrete (whichever is less), psi,

and f_c = minimum allowable compressive strength of the strata rock or concrete (whichever is less), psi.

The designer should consider that the values of f_s and f_c obtained from sampling might not conservatively represent the strength of the destressed edges of the coal pillars. Further, the designer should select a required length based on the larger of the values obtained from Equations 10 and 11. In addition, a factor of safety at least equal to 2 should then be applied to the required length. Equations 10 and 11 are most applicable to high head situations where the resulting bulkhead acts as a massive plug. If they indicate a relatively narrow bulkhead, i.e., a bulkhead with a thickness-to-height ratio less than 1.0, then the bulkhead would need to be checked for adequate flexural strength.

Methods of increasing the resistance along the interface include notching the bulkheads into the surrounding strata, tapering the plug, and/or installing epoxy-coated (corrosion-resistant) dowel rods into the strata and allowing the rods to protrude into the bulkhead material. The dowel rods should have an embedded length into the strata and into the bulkhead sufficient to develop the strength of the dowel rod without having a bond failure.

Large mass plugs should have at least minimal temperature and shrinkage steel placed in accordance with ACI 207.2R, "Cracking of Mass Concrete" [ACI 1995].

Shear Design of Reinforced Concrete Bulkheads

While the above equations can be used to evaluate the shear strength of the long bulkhead plugs, for thinner reinforced concrete bulkheads the following expressions can be used to calculate the concrete's design shear strength:

$$V_c = \Phi 2\sqrt{f'_c}\, b_w d \tag{12}$$

where V_c = shear strength of the concrete bulkhead per unit width, lb,
                  Φ = 0.75 (shear strength reduction factor),
                  f'_c = compressive strength of concrete, psi,
                  b_w = unit width of bulkhead (12 in),

and d = distance from extreme compression fiber to centroid of tension reinforcement, in.

If the above expression indicates inadequate concrete shear strength, there is a more rigorous and exact expression found in ACI 318, section 11.3. In addition, the contribution of steel reinforcement (ACI 318, section 11.5) could be added to the value obtained for the concrete to get a combined strength for the member.

For thick reinforced concrete bulkheads where the ratio of the clear span distance (l_n, in) to the depth (d, in) from the waterside of the bulkhead to the centroid of the tensile steel reinforcement is less than 4, section 11.8 of ACI 318 should be applied. As indicated above, it should be noted that the span-to-depth ratios are different for shear design than for flexural design.

If lightweight concrete with densities of 100–110 lb/ft^3 are used, the values of V_c obtained using $\sqrt{f_c}$ in the expression should be multiplied by 0.75 for "all lightweight" concrete and by 0.85 for "sand-lightweight" concrete, per section 11.2 of ACI 318 [MSHA and OSM 2003].

> **The bulkhead must be able to resist the shear and bending stresses acting on it with a safety factor consistent with the degree of uncertainty and the consequences of failure.**

Cement Selection

During the curing of a large mass of confined concrete such as a plug, cracking and shrinkage can occur. For this reason, prolonged and thorough curing is a significant factor in attaining impermeable, watertight concrete. Cracking is usually caused by high heat of hydration generated during curing. This weakens the concrete and may affect its ability to resist a design pressure. Shrinkage can affect anchorage at the perimeter and is a result of excessive water content or inadequate aggregate composition. Some shrinkage is inevitable in concrete, and pressure grouting is necessary to improve contact between the bulkhead and surrounding rock. The addition of pozzolans, such as fly ash, to concrete can improve workability, reduce heat of hydration and shrinkage, and increase resistance to sulfates contained in water. However, caution must be exercised in selecting pozzolans because their properties vary widely and excessive amounts may have adverse effects on the concrete such as increased shrinkage and reduced strength and durability [U.S. Bureau of Reclamation 1975]. Before selecting a mix, trial mixes should be made, especially when using admixtures and pozzolans.

To attain concrete with specific properties, other types of portland cement can be used. Type II is for general use, more specifically, when moderate sulfate resistance and heat of hydration are desired. Type IV gives a low heat of hydration, and Type V is used when high sulfate resistance is desired (see Table 3). Standard specifications for portland cement are given in ASTM Standard C150 [ASTM 2007]. Standard specifications for coal fly ash and raw or calcined natural pozzolan for use in concrete are given in ASTM Standard C618 [ASTM 2005; Chekan 1985].

The following details the eight types of portland cement from ASTM C150 that are available for bulkhead construction [ASTM 2007].

23

- Type I: For use when the special properties specified for any other type are not required.
- Type IA: Air-entraining cement for the same uses as Type I, where air entrainment is desired.
- Type II: For general use, more especially, when moderate sulfate resistance or moderate heat of hydration is desired.
- Type IIA: Air-entraining cement for the same uses as Type II, where air entrainment is desired.
- Type III: For use when high early strength is desired.
- Type IIIA: Air-entraining cement for the same uses as Type III where air entrainment is desired.
- Type IV: For use when low heat of hydration is desired.
- Type V: For use when high sulfate resistance is desired.

Table 3.—Attack on concrete by soils and waters containing various sulfate concentrations
[U.S. Bureau of Reclamation 1975]

Relative degree of sulfate attack	Sulfate (as SO_4) in water samples, ppm	Cement type
Negligible	0–150	I
Moderate	150–1,500	II
Severe	1,500–10,000	V
Very severe	10,000 or more	V plus pozzolan

When concrete is used in the construction of bulkheads, the type selected should be based on the sulfate concentration of the fluid impounded and the heat of hydration desired.

Conduits Passing Through Bulkheads

Conduits passing through the bulkheads are commonly used for monitoring head pressure, the atmosphere within the sealed area, or for providing a means to control the fluid level within the impoundment. They must be designed to prevent failure from overpressure, blockage, and seepage along the interface of the conduit and bulkhead. Details and drawings of how the installation will address these requirements must be submitted in the permit application. The following guidelines will assist the designer in this task.

- Select conduit material that is capable of withstanding at least four times the maximum head pressure created from the impounded fluid or ventilation requirements and capable of conveying the anticipated flow.

- Select conduit material that is corrosion-resistant, such as polyvinyl chloride (PVC) or high-density polyethylene. Steel or other conduit material that is able to conduct electricity may not be permitted for installations that serve as ventilation seals.

- Install a strainer or screen on the fluid side of the monitoring conduits to prevent blockage from sediment.

- Estimate the anticipated inflow fluid rate, and install conduits of the proper size and quantity to reduce the fluid level of the impoundment. Incorporate trash racks or other screened devices on the fluid side of these conduits to prevent blockage.

- Equip monitoring lines with a means to back-flush the conduit. This can be accomplished by installing an auxiliary port with a shutoff valve on the fresh-air side of the conduit. Water pressure or compressed air that exceeds the head pressure can be used to back-flush the line.

- Install antiseep collars on all conduits passing through the bulkhead to prevent leakage between the conduit and bulkhead.

Conduits passing through the bulkhead must be of adequate size for the anticipated pressure and flow rates, be corrosion-resistant, and use antiseep collars to prevent leakage at the conduit/bulkhead interface.

Method to Control Fluid Elevation

Controlling the fluid level in the impoundment is essential for safe operation. Some locations allow the water/slurry to overflow into another area once it reaches a certain elevation, which in turn limits the pressure on the bulkhead. Others require surface or underground pumps to control the fluid elevation. The permit package will require details of how the fluid elevation will be maintained. Keep in mind that regulations may prohibit the direct connection of an electrical pump to a conduit that extends into an abandoned area. The details should include the following:

- The planned minimum and maximum fluid elevations

- Estimate of the fluid quantity impounded at minimum and maximum elevations

- Details of the pumping system, if required, to maintain pool elevation, such as:
  - Location and size of pumps
  - Planned pumping rates and pumping schedule
  - Location of electrical controls
  - Monitoring of pump performance
  - Contingency plan if pump failure occurs
  - Plans to control pool elevation during anticipated outages

- Calculations to confirm that the pumping system or overflow discharge capacity of the impoundment is adequately sized to handle the anticipated peak inflow rate of fluid. Include consideration for seasonal variations.

- Installation of corrosion-resistant flow-through pipes with gate valves on the outby side of each bulkhead for emergency drawdown. Include calculations confirming that these flow-through pipes are able to discharge fluid at a rate that exceeds the anticipated inflow rate. Also include a map indicating the fluid flow path if the pipes are used to reduce the impoundment level.

- Where applicable, a fluid flow path for systems that allows the impoundment to overflow into other sections of the mine.

- For fluid retention systems that discharge directly to surface areas through mine openings or open conduits, provisions to restrict access to the underground mine through the opening or conduit.

For bulkhead installations that do not act as ventilation seals, an acceptable means of preventing the pool from exceeding maximum elevation is to install a corrosion-resistant pressure relief valve(s) or rupture disc(s) on one or more of the bulkheads. These devices require installing an upstream valve to cut off the flow should the disc rupture or the relief valve open. If one of these options is selected, document that the expected flow path fluid will travel if the disc ruptures or the relief valve opens. Also, ensure that the force from fluid discharging out of the valve or disc will not severely erode the surrounding strata.

> **Install corrosion-resistant flow-through pipes with gate valves on the outby side of each bulkhead for emergency drawdown of the impoundment.**

Leakage Prevention

Fluid can escape from an underground impoundment at the bulkhead location along three paths: through the surrounding strata, at the interface of the bulkhead and strata, and directly through the bulkhead. Leakage through the strata is discussed earlier in the "Geotechnical Considerations" section, with suggestions for restricting this pathway.

At the interface of the bulkhead and surrounding strata, it is not uncommon for voids to develop. This is due to shrinkage during the cure period for concrete or from improperly placed bulkhead construction material. This is especially problematic for thinner bulkheads. Regardless of how they develop, procedures must be detailed in the permit package for controlling this leakage path.

Contact grouting is a widely used method for filling voids at the interface. Placing steel pipe or packers at predetermined locations along the concrete/strata interface before the concrete is poured usually provides holes for contact grouting. The pipes, which protrude from the forms, act as a travelway for the grout after the concrete cures. At times, during the pouring of the bulkhead, the pipe may fill with concrete, which must then be drilled out so that grout can migrate properly along the interface [Chekan 1985].

> **Contact grouting of the interface of the bulkhead and surrounding strata should be conducted on all long-term bulkhead installations.**

Bulkheads that are constructed from a continuous pour of material are not prone to leakage through the structure unless heat created as the material cures causes fractures or joints in the base material. When cementitious material is used to construct the bulkhead, the heat of hydration must be controlled (see ACI 207.2R, "Cracking of Mass Concrete" [ACI 1995]). If required, select a concrete type with low heat of hydration (see "Cement Selection" section above) and, if necessary, make provisions to install cooling tubes in the bulkhead and include procedures to grout close the cooling tubes when no longer needed. When structures are constructed in layers, make provisions to mitigate cracking between lifts.

> **Make provisions to control the heat of hydration when using cementitious materials by selecting the proper concrete placement schedule and using cooling tubes.**

Emergency Response Plan

All efforts must be made to design the fluid retention system in such a manner that failure will not occur. However, changes in strata conditions, structural failure, excessive rainfall, impact from abandoned works, and various other conditions could trigger an emergency response. Early in the permit documentation, plan for employee evacuation if failure of the fluid retention system occurs. In developing an Emergency Response Plan, consider the path fluid would flow based on mine floor elevations and determine possible areas requiring evacuation. If escaping fluid will discharge to the surface, consider the locations on the surface that must be evacuated. The Emergency Response Plan should detail what steps will be taken in the event that fluid leakage from the impoundment becomes significant, fluid elevation in the impoundment changes unexpectedly, and/or fluid level increases significantly beyond the normal operating elevation.

A common method is to develop a plan based on a list of actions to be taken when the normal pool elevation is exceeded. At one of the mining operations visited by NIOSH researchers, the Emergency Plan is initiated when the normal pool elevation is exceeded by 10 ft. This requires an increase in the bulkhead inspection frequency from weekly to daily and requires the employees be notified of the situation. If the normal pool elevation is exceeded by 15 ft, the inspection frequency is increased to hourly and the mine is evacuated of all nonessential employees. If the pool elevation is exceeded by 20 ft, the mine is evacuated. This particular operation electronically monitors the head pressure on the bulkhead through the mine monitoring system and has the ability to monitor the fluid level in the impoundment from the surface via boreholes into the impoundment area. The operation also uses deep well pumps to control fluid levels in the impoundment, which allows the fluid level to be lowered without the presence of personnel underground.

The Emergency Response Plan should detail what actions are to be taken if certain events occur, such as exceeding normal head pressure, failure of pumping systems that control the impoundment fluid level, power outages, seismic activity, excessive leakage, and/or increased leakage without increase in head pressure. Examine the operation, develop a list of the events that could impact the bulkhead system, and determine what action should be taken if these events occur.

Each operation has the potential for specific events that could negatively impact the operation of the fluid retention system. When developing the Emergency Response Plan, discuss these issues with personnel who are familiar with the daily mining operations and develop a list of events that would impact the proposed impoundment. Some common events are:

- Electrical interruptions
- Mechanical failures of the pumping and discharge system
- Exceptionally high fluid inflow related to seasonal variations
- Increased leakage in the bulkhead area without increase in head pressure
- Deterioration of roof conditions
- Seismic activity
- Fluid leakage through barrier pillars
- Deterioration of coal pillars supporting the bulkhead
- Bulkhead failure

To initiate an emergency response, a list of specific events is required to initiate specific required action. These include the following:

- Fluid level in the impoundment exceeds normal operation level by a specified amount
- Force exerted on the bulkhead by fluid in the impoundment exceeds a specified maximum pressure
- Increased leakage through strata or bulkhead not associated with an increase in head pressure
- Measured or perceived movement of the bulkhead
- Deterioration of roof conditions that prevents routine inspections
- Deterioration of roof or floor conditions that could impact the structural integrity of the bulkhead
- Indications that piping is occurring along the bulkhead or strata interface
- Explosive gas mixtures behind the bulkheads before impounding fluids are at or above the roof level in the abandoned area

Next, determine what emergency response is required for each event. Some common actions include the following:

- Increase monitoring of bulkheads.
- Notify personnel.
- Evacuate people in the area that could be inundated if failure occurs.
- Evacuate all people not required to maintain the mine and monitor bulkheads.
- Complete evacuation of the mine.
- Start up additional pumps.
- Open valves on flow-through discharge pipes.
- Start notification of mine management officials.
- Start notification of regulatory agencies.

The Emergency Response Plan should include a list of people and agencies that are to be notified when specific events occur. The list should include primary and secondary people to contact with their work, home, and cell phone numbers. The list should be broken down into groups that are to be notified depending on the urgency of the situation. Some common departments, agencies, and people to contact are:

- Mine operations

    - Mine manager, superintendent, etc.
    - Mine foreman and shift foreman
    - Safety Department
    - Maintenance Department
    - Engineering Department
    - Human Resources

- Agencies

    - MSHA
    - State mining agency
    - State environmental agency
    - Local emergency response coordinator
    - Local and State Police
    - Local Fire Department
    - Local ambulance squad

- Other

    - Pump manufacturer

The Emergency Response Plan is valuable only if employees are trained in the procedures and can carry out their responsibilities when an emergency occurs. A training program must be developed for the fluid retention system and incorporated into the routine and refresher training schedule and safety talks for the operation. The plan should cover the basic operation of the system, events that would require action, appropriate responses, and evacuation plans and procedures.

> **The Emergency Response Plan must include provisions for routine and refresher training of all employees at the operation. Training must include procedures to follow, areas of responsibility, and evacuation plans and travel routes.**

Summary

- Bulkheads installed across mine entries may seal off abandoned mine works. Mine ventilation seals must be able to withstand explosion pressures of at least 50 or 120 psi, depending on the installation. A registered professional engineer with a strong background in structural design and a working knowledge of underground mining operations must design these structures.

- The installation of an underground impoundment must not pose a safety threat to the workforce. The impoundment must be located at an elevation that will not trap miners and prevent their escape to the surface if a breach occurs and have reserve capacity to accommodate periods when fluid cannot be removed.

- An evaluation must be conducted to confirm that the bulkhead is being placed in competent rock at a site that will remain stable for the life of the impoundment. A trained professional that has experience in performing this type of site assessment must conduct this evaluation.

- To ensure the stability of the bulkheads and the strata supporting the impoundment, mining underlying works in the vicinity of the underground fluid retention system should be minimized.

- The bulkhead must be designed to withstand the static pressure exerted by the maximum impounded fluid level with consideration for ventilation seal requirements, seismic loading, and an acceptable margin of safety.

- The geology of the strata surrounding the impoundment must be tested and determined to be adequate for construction of an impoundment.

- Concrete is widely used to construct bulkheads. The concrete selected must be based on the chemistry of the fluid impounded and the heat of hydration desired.

- Ring grouting should be conducted to control fluid leakage through the strata, and contact pressure grouting should be performed to control leakage at the bulkhead/ strata interface.

- An Emergency Response Plan must be developed that provides for the safe evacuation of all underground employees in the event that an emergency develops related to the operation of the underground fluid retention system.

CONSTRUCTION

Although many of the construction details and requirements are outlined in the permit package, a section detailing the construction procedures for the bulkheads is required. Include information and plans that cover preconstruction site preparation through to the completion and turnover of the fluid retention system.

Site Preparation

The work area and travel routes for accessing the site must be cleared of debris and made safe for travel of employees. Roadways required for transporting material and equipment must be surveyed to determine height and width restrictions for transported materials and to confirm that adequate storage areas are accessible. The following is a list of common activities associated with underground site preparation. The permit package should include a drawing or mine map to designate where these activities will be conducted and other planned site preparation work.

- Scaling roof and ribs
- Cleanup of loose coal and rock in work areas and haulage routes
- Replacement of existing roof support, where required
- Installation of additional roof support, where required
- Removal of excess water from construction site and haulage routes
- Removal of weak, degradable floor material
- Excavation of keyways or notches into the mine strata
- Designation of material storage areas
- Rock dust application

Construction Techniques

The actual construction and installation of the bulkhead may be conducted by mine personnel or contract workers. In either case, a written plan is required that specifies the phases of construction and details how the work will be accomplished. Some of the more common items to include are the following:

- Method and procedures for trenching roof, rib, and floor (if required), including any preconstruction requirements. Some installations require installing steel angles that are rock bolted into the strata along the floor/bulkhead and roof/bulkhead intersection in place of hitching.

- Form construction:[7]

  ○ Include detailed drawings that specify dimensions, material list, anchorage details, and assembly and construction procedures.
  ○ Include calculations verifying that the forms are properly designed to resist the hydraulic head of the construction material as it is placed and cures.

- When concrete block walls are to be used as forms, specify:

  ○ Type and size of block used, minimum compressive strength required, and mortar or bonding agent
  ○ Method or procedures to keep the wall plumb and level
  ○ Method or procedure to tighten or wedge the wall against the strata
  ○ If walls are to be removed once the bulkhead material cures to enhance inspections
  ○ When surface coatings are used, give specific details including the manufacturer and type, along with application guidelines and procedures.

---

[7]ACI 347–04, "Guide to Formwork for Concrete" [ACI 2004], may provide useful information for this section.

- Detail drawings for placement of reinforcement bars with the following information:
  - Specifications for reinforcement bars including size, yield strength, and coating requirements
  - Procedures for anchoring the reinforcement bars into the surrounding strata. Specify the size, depth, location, and spacing of holes, along with specifications and procedures for grouting the reinforcement bars into the strata.
  - Acceptable methods to join sections of reinforcement bars
  - If mechanical couplings are used, specify the type and minimum strength requirements.
- Describe procedure for mixing or blending bulkhead construction material:
  - Include details of the required formulation and required timeframe for material placement in the forms.
  - Specify machine or equipment needed to blend or mix material.
  - List any special handling procedures, safety precautions, and personal protective equipment (PPE) required.
- Detail placement of bulkhead construction material from blending or mixing equipment to the form:
  - Describe route material will travel.
  - List device used to pump or pneumatically stow the material.
  - List methods or procedures used to ensure proper placement of the material within the forms.
  - Detail procedures to follow if cold joints occur (planned or unplanned) during placement of the material.
  - Specify required curing period for material used.

> **Develop a detailed construction plan for each construction phase of the underground fluid retention system. This should cover initial site preparation through startup of the installation.**

Training

All personnel involved in constructing the fluid retention system should be given an overview of the project and made aware of the specific hazards associated with the installation and startup of the system. In addition, plan for routine safety talks to review safety procedures and spot safety talks to discuss safety issues or situations that develop during the installation. Some topics that should be covered with all personnel include:

- Operation of mobile equipment
- Review of material safety data sheets (MSDSs) for the construction materials used
- Review of site-specific hazards and safe work practices
- Modifications or additions to existing roof control measures
- Required PPE
- Primary and secondary escapeway routes

> **The construction plan must include provisions for properly training all employees involved in installing the underground fluid retention system.**

Quality Control Plan

A written quality control plan is required to ensure that the installation meets or exceeds the parameters used in designing the underground impoundment. The plan should detail monitoring the material supplied for the installation, construction procedures, and steps to follow if substandard work or materials are encountered. All products or material used for constructing and installing the bulkhead system should be monitored to ensure that they meet the design criteria and are installed or placed in the manner prescribed by the designer. Designate specific personnel to monitor quality or performance, and specify their areas of responsibility.

- Develop a material list for the project that includes the parameters to be monitored. Include maximum and minimum acceptable levels when possible.

- Develop a plan for where material is to be stored both underground and on the surface. Include any special requirements for each product, such as hazardous storage, allowable temperature range, exposure to sunlight, low moisture, etc.

- Develop a plan for transportation from the vendor to the mine site and from the surface to underground location. Include any special handling requirements.

- Include PPE requirements for handling materials.

> **Develop a material handling plan for the project. Include a list of all required materials, transportation and storage plan, special handling procedures, and required PPE.**

Although the material may have already passed initial quality control, followup should be conducted by the field monitor for:

- Damaged packaging that may render the material unacceptable

- Damage to material that occurred during transportation from the surface to underground location

- Any material that is delivered directly to the construction site that did not pass through quality control

- Monitoring of material placement should be outlined in the plan and procedures for documentation of this work. Also, include procedures to follow if the prescribed procedure cannot be followed due to field conditions.

- Material formulated on-site such as concrete or polyurethane foam will require field testing to verify compliance with the design specifications. The tests must be conducted at a certified testing facility and follow ASTM standards. The plan should cover the number of samples to be taken per yard, per load, or lift, the acceptable range of field test results, the acceptable range of laboratory test results, and should include a paper trail to ensure that the correct samples are properly tested. Also include the procedure to follow if substandard material is discovered.

- The construction supervisor should maintain a detailed log of daily construction activities. The log should include sketches and photos that document field conditions, material issues, and procedures followed.

> **Develop a detailed quality control program for monitoring the installation of the underground fluid retention system that ensures that the raw materials meet design specifications, proper construction techniques are followed, required testing is performed, and both written and photographic documentation is provided.**

Summary

- A detailed construction plan must be developed for each construction phase of the underground fluid retention system. The plan must include provisions for training employees on material handling procedures, required PPE, MSDS information, equipment operation, and general underground mine safety.

- Material handling plans and procedures should be developed for the project. This includes a list of all required materials, transportation and storage plans, and special handling procedures.

- A detailed quality control program must be instituted for monitoring the installation of the underground fluid retention system. This will help ensure that raw materials meet design specifications, proper construction techniques are followed, required testing is performed, and both written and photographic documentation is logged for future reference.

MONITORING

The basic requirement for monitoring an underground fluid retention system is to conduct routine examinations of the bulkheads and surrounding strata. The examiner should look for signs of increased stress or deterioration of the bulkhead material, visually inspect the surrounding strata from the bulkhead to and including the outby crosscut for signs of piping, examine for leakage and changes in the condition of the strata, and measure the leakage rate and head pressure. All information gathered during the inspection should be recorded in a logbook designated for that purpose and countersigned by mine management. The following subjects should be addressed in the permit package.

Routine Inspections

Bulkhead systems should be inspected at least once per week. More frequent routine inspections are recommended for systems that have the potential to inundate active mine works. Other factors that would indicate additional inspections are needed include:

- Unexpected increase in head pressure at the structure
- Head pressure increases beyond expected maximum
- Increased fluid inflow due to seasonal changes
- Increased leakage rates without corresponding change in head pressure
- Increased concentrated leakage at any one area
- Noted changes in the strata that could affect the integrity of the bulkhead system

State and federal agencies may require more frequent inspections. Contact these agencies for guidance before submitting the permit application.

To assist the examiner, develop a checklist for documenting head pressures, leakage rates, pump performance information, and conditions of the bulkhead and strata observed during the inspection. Also allow for additional observations such as leakage around conduits passing through the bulkhead or at the interface of the bulkhead and strata. A sample inspection sheet is shown in Appendix B.

> **Develop an impoundment inspection checklist report tailored to the installation to document operating pressures, changes in strata, leakage rates, and signs of weakness.**

Head Pressure

Bulkhead installations require a device to accurately monitor the hydrostatic head applied by the impounded fluid. By far, the most common method of meeting this requirement is to install a quality pressure gauge on a conduit passing through the bulkhead with the lowest elevation into the fluid. The pressure indicated by the gauge is the value recorded during the routine inspections. This method is recommended as the primary method to monitor head pressure because it does not require a power source to generate information.

A secondary system that continuously monitors bulkhead pressure is recommended. At operations that employ mine monitoring systems, an electronic pressure transducer can be mounted on the bulkhead with the lowest floor elevation. The transducer is connected to the mine monitoring system, which continuously monitors and records the bulkhead pressure. The mine monitoring systems normally display in areas that are manned around the clock and will set off an alarm if the preset pressure is exceeded. At operations that do not have mine monitoring systems, data logging devices can be used to document the pressure loading of the bulkhead. These devices can be set up to trigger an alarm if a specified pressure is exceeded.

It is understood that bulkheads installed in return air courses may not be able to use electronic devices to monitor head pressure. It is recommended that pressure transducers be installed on more than one bulkhead to provide a backup source for monitoring head pressures.

At installations where it is anticipated that the fluid level will not exceed the height of the bulkhead, a visual level indicator can be installed.

For impoundments that cannot be monitored underground, surface monitoring wells must be established to track fluid levels. A cased borehole or other conduit that provides access from the surface to the impoundment fluid and of suitable diameter to accommodate a piezometer or similar device can be used determine the fluid elevation. Surface monitoring wells should also be considered to provide a backup means of determining the fluid level of an underground impoundment when access into the mine is not permitted.

> **If possible, install an electronic pressure transducer to monitor the head pressure on the bulkhead system. This device should be connected to a data recording system that logs head pressure and can trigger an alarm if a specified pressure is exceeded.**
>
> **Provide backup methods or procedures to determine the fluid level in the impoundment.**

Pump Performance

Operations that use pumping systems to maintain the fluid level should make provisions to monitor the inflow and outflow rates of the fluid retention system. This may not be possible at all installations due to fluid that free flows from adjacent mine works into the impoundment area, but operations that use pumps to add and remove fluid from the impoundment can monitor the performance of the pumps, which can provide information to calculate the amount of fluid passing through the impoundment. By recording the pumping times, pump speed, and discharge pressures and calculating the system losses, the volume of fluid handled by a pump can be determined. Information from this monitoring is useful in determining efficiency of the pumping system and the ability to handle additional fluid.

> **Develop a system to monitor the inflow and outflow rates of the underground fluid retention system.**

Drainage and Monitoring Pipes

On the impoundment side, drainage and monitoring pipe inlets must be protected to prevent debris from blocking the entrance. This can be accomplished by installing trash racks, screens, or filters. Monitoring pipes must be equipped with shutoff valves to allow for change-out of gauges and pressure transducers, and spare or duplicate monitoring pipes should be installed in at least one other bulkhead.

Leakage

During the design phase, make provisions to monitor leakage of the bulkhead system. This will help generate a performance curve, i.e., static water head at the bulkhead versus leakage rate. A simple method to monitor leakage is to install a low water dam outby the bulkhead and monitor the amount of water passing through a triangular weir. It is recommended that leakage be monitored from each bulkhead separately. If this is not possible, allow the leakage to flow to a central gathering point, and build the low water dam with a triangular weir at that location.

> **Provide a method to monitor leakage rates from the underground fluid retention system.**

Deflection

Electronic devices are available to monitor deflection of the bulkhead due to convergence or pressure loading. The instruments commonly used to measure the displacements include vibrating wire strain gauges, linear variable displacement transducers (LVDTs), and potentiometers. These devices can be connected to mine monitoring systems or data loggers to provide continuous monitoring of the displacements. The bulkhead displacement that would normally be of most interest in evaluating bulkhead behavior is the horizontal deflection. However, roof-to-floor convergence can be measured to determine if ground movement is causing bulkhead loading or to determine if there are ground stability issues in the vicinity of the bulkhead. The measured displacements can then be plotted against time to determine if the bulkhead is stable or against the pressure head to determine the response of the bulkhead to load and load changes. These devices may not be permitted for bulkheads installed in return air courses.

Summary

- An inspection checklist should be developed to log information from routine inspections. The checklist should be site-specific and document head pressures observed, changes in strata, and leakage rates and should note any conditions that indicate signs of weakness of the installation. A sample inspection sheet is shown in Appendix B.

- A visual pressure gauge is the most common and acceptable method of monitoring the head pressure exerted on a bulkhead. Systems that continuously monitor and record the head pressure at the bulkhead and go into alarm mode if a specified pressure is recorded are available and should be installed where conditions permit.

- It is important to monitor the inflow and discharge rates of the fluid retention system. Using flow meters and recording pump operating times, pump speed, and discharge pressures will provide information to calculate the volume of fluid handled. This information is useful in determining efficiency of the pumping system and the ability to handle additional fluid, if needed.

- Leakage monitoring should be provided for in the bulkhead system design and is necessary to evaluate the performance of the system. Plotting the leakage rate against the head pressure will determine if leakage is increasing due to increased head pressure or because additional leakage pathways are developing.

- Electronic devices are available for installations that plan to monitor deflection of the bulkhead due to convergence or pressure loading. Instruments that can perform this task include vibrating wire strain gauges, LVDTs, and potentiometers. These devices must be connected to mine monitoring systems or data loggers to continuously record the information.

CONCLUSIONS

NIOSH researchers, with assistance from MSHA, conducted an extensive review of bulkhead permits and visited accessible bulkhead installations at underground mining operations to gather information related to permitting procedures, construction practices, maintenance issues, monitoring procedures, and Emergency Response Plans. The study indicated that once the need for an underground fluid retention structure was identified, considerable engineering hours were spent designing bulkheads, but less effort was placed on addressing the reaction of the surrounding strata to the impoundment, future mine plans, long-term ground control, monitoring systems, and emergency response. Discussions with mine operators, consulting engineers, and permit reviewers indicated a lack of available information to assist them in preparing the proper permitting package for an underground fluid retention system.

While conducting this research, NIOSH determined that the underground impoundment and bulkheads should be permitted and designed as a system with consideration given for how the bulkheads interact with the strata and fluid handling system controlling the fluid level in the impoundment. This approach identified the following guidelines that must be considered:

- Bulkheads that also function as mine ventilation seals may have increased strength requirements. These bulkhead designs and related calculations must be performed by a registered professional engineer with a strong background in structural design and a working knowledge of underground mining operations.

- Safety of the mine personnel and the ability to evacuate the mine are paramount to the design. The impoundment must be located at an elevation that will not trap miners and prevent their escape to the surface if a breach occurs.

- Over the life of the impoundment, power interruptions will occur and mechanical repairs will be required. The fluid retention system should have a built-in reserve capacity to allow for situations or conditions that prevent the removal of fluid from the impoundment.

- Consideration must be given to sources of fluid from adjacent mine works that could enter the proposed impoundment. Identify all mine works, both active and inactive, that could impact the amount of fluid flowing into and out of the proposed underground impoundment.

- It must be demonstrated that the bulkhead is being placed in competent rock at a site that will remain stable for the life of the impoundment. This evaluation must be conducted by a trained professional with experience in performing this type of site assessment.

- Strata directly in contact with the bulkhead should have a slake durability index of at least medium-high, and the CMRR immersion test results should be in the slightly to not-sensitive categories.

- Engineering calculations demonstrating that the coal pillars to which the bulkheads are anchored have a sufficient safety factor for long-term stability must be provided.

- Leakage through the strata and at the bulkhead/strata interface must be controlled. Ring grouting of the strata around the bulkhead and contact grouting of the bulkhead/strata interface are recommended.

- Measures must be taken to ensure that the roof remains stable at the bulkhead locations to prevent development of leakage paths through the strata. Installing additional roof support on both sides of the bulkheads must be considered.

- The strata surrounding the bulkhead must be strong enough to support the structure. Remove immediate roof or floor material from the footprint of the bulkhead that is affected by water, damaged, or fractured by mining.

- To maintain the integrity of the strata supporting the underground fluid retention system, avoid mining underlying works in the vicinity of the bulkheads or the impoundment.

- Reinforced concrete structures should be designed in accordance with the most recent versions of ACI 318 and 350.

- Nonreinforced concrete structures should be designed so that the resistance of the structure is at least two times the force from the external loading.

- The bulkhead must be designed to withstand the maximum pressure that could be exerted on the structure. To determine this value, consider exterior sources of water or fluid that could enter the impoundment area through the coal seam or surrounding strata.

- At many locations, bulkheads function as mine ventilation seals. These installations may be required to meet current federal regulations governing ventilation seals.

- The permit package must include calculations confirming that the barrier pillar is of sufficient width to support the roof and maintain the separation between the impoundment and other existing or projected workings.

- Concrete is commonly used in the construction of bulkheads. When concrete is used, the type selected must be based on the sulfate concentration of the fluid impounded and the desired heat of hydration.

- Conduits passing through the bulkhead will be required to monitor head pressure and emergency drawdown of the impoundment. These conduits must be adequately sized for the anticipated pressures and flow rates, be corrosion-resistant, and use antiseep collars to prevent leakage at the conduit/bulkhead interface. The emergency drawdown conduits must be equipped with gate valves on the outby side of the bulkhead.

- When concrete is poured in large quantities, heat of hydration must be controlled. If the selected bulkhead design requires large quantities of concrete, make provisions to control the heat of hydration by selecting the proper concrete and using cooling tubes. The cooling tubes must be completely filled with grout when no longer required.

- An Emergency Response Plan must be developed that provides for the safe evacuation of all affected personnel if a breach of the impoundment occurs. The plan must be routinely reviewed with all employees at the operation.

- A detailed construction plan for each phase of the underground fluid retention system should be developed. This should cover initial site preparation through startup of the installation. The construction plan must also include provisions for training all employees involved in installing the underground fluid retention system.

- A plan to transport, handle, and store material necessary for constructing the underground impoundment should be developed. The plan should include a list of all required materials, transportation procedures, location of storage areas, special handling procedures, and required PPE.

- A detailed quality control program for monitoring the installation of the underground fluid retention system must be developed. The plan should ensure that the raw materials meet design specifications, proper construction techniques are followed, required testing is performed, and written and photographic documentation is obtained.

- Routine monitoring of the bulkheads will be required. Develop an impoundment inspection and checklist report tailored to the installation to document operating pressures, changes in strata, leakage rates, and signs of weakness. A sample inspection sheet is shown in Appendix B.

- A pressure gauge for visually monitoring the head pressure on the bulkhead will be required. The gauge should be installed with a shutoff valve to isolate the head pressure during gauge replacement.

- Continuous monitoring and recording of the bulkhead is recommended. If possible, install an electronic pressure transducer to monitor the head pressure on the bulkhead system. This device should be connected to a data recording system that logs head pressure and has the ability to trigger an alarm if the head pressure exceeds preset levels.

- Consideration should be given to providing a means of determining the fluid level in the impoundment when access to the mine is prohibited.

- Pumps are routinely used to control the fluid level of the impoundment. Monitoring the performance of these pumps is recommended to determine the efficiency of the underground impoundment and the amount of fluid being pumped.

- Leakage in the vicinity of the bulkheads is not uncommon and should be monitored. A system or method should be incorporated into the system design to monitor this leakage.

The guidelines in this report are intended to be used as a framework for developing and permitting a safe and efficient underground fluid retention system that will remain stable for the life of the impoundment. Although this report has identified many of the key areas to address and common design considerations, the guidelines should not be considered all-encompassing. It would be nearly impossible to list all of the features, situations, and conditions that could impact the integrity of each and every underground impoundment. Therefore, the responsibility of identifying these site-specific conditions rests with the permit applicant.

ACKNOWLEDGMENTS

The authors thank the following members of the mining community for the opportunity to visit their operations and discuss issues related to underground impoundments: Terry Savage, General Mine Foreman, and Horace J. (Jody) Theriot III, Manager of Human Resources and Safety, Mettiki Coal, Oakland, MD; Dennis L. Chiari, Ventilation Engineer, and Edward Sartain, Safety Supervisor, Shoal Creek Mine, Drummond Coal, Inc., Jasper, AL; Greg Patterson, General Manager, No. 18 Mine, Long Branch Energy, Danville, WV; Donnie Pauley, Safety Manager, Peabody Coal Co., Van, WV; Charles L. Lilly, P.E., P.S., Director of Engineering, Patriot Coal Corp., Henderson, KY; and Keith Brown, Senior Engineer, formerly with Highland Mining Co., Henderson, KY.

The authors also thank the following regulatory personnel for their assistance in gathering information on existing and proposed bulkhead installations: Kelvin K. Wu, Ph.D., Chief (now retired), Mine Waste and Geotechnical Engineering Division, MSHA Technical Support, Pittsburgh, PA; Theodore P. (Pat) Betoney, Mining/Civil Engineer (now retired), and Bunie Harper, Civil Engineer (now retired), MSHA District 3, Morgantown, WV; Harold Owens, Supervisor–Impoundments, MSHA District 4, Mount Hope, WV; Ronnie Joe Dooley, Supervisor–Coal Mine Safety and Health Inspector, MSHA District 4, Madison Subdistrict, Madison, WV; Robert "Hank" Bellamy, Mining Engineer, MSHA District 6, Pikeville, KY; Lewis Stanley, Supervisor–Ventilation (now retired), and Sarah A. (Alice) Perry, Mining Engineer, MSHA District 10, Madisonville, KY; Jackie Shubert, Ventilation Specialist, and Stephen Harrison, Ventilation Specialist, MSHA District 11, Birmingham, AL; William Bookshar, Engineering Supervisor, and Thomas McKnight, P.E., Mining Engineer 2, Pennsylvania Bureau of Deep Mine Safety, Uniontown, PA; and Monte Hieb, Chief Engineer, West Virginia Office of Miners' Health, Safety, and Training, Oak Hill, WV.

In addition, the authors acknowledge the following NIOSH Pittsburgh Research Laboratory personnel without whose contributions this project could not have been accomplished: Michael J. Sapko, Senior Scientist (now retired), for his insight in developing the project and technical assistance; Stephen C. Tadolini, Branch Chief, Rock Safety Engineering Branch, for his direction in the project and providing resources; Eric S. Weiss, Team Leader, Lake Lynn Laboratory, for his assistance in gathering field data; and Gerrit V. R. Goodman, Team Leader, Ventilation and Explosion Prevention Section, Disaster Prevention and Response Branch, for his assistance and guidance in developing the final report.

REFERENCES

72 Fed. Reg. 28795 [2007]. Mine Safety and Health Administration, 30 CFR part 75: sealing of abandoned areas; emergency temporary standard.

ACI (American Concrete Institute) [1995]. Cracking of mass concrete (207.2R). Farmington Hills, MI: American Concrete Institute.

ACI (American Concrete Institute) [2004]. Guide to formwork for concrete (347–04). Farmington Hills, MI: American Concrete Institute.

ACI (American Concrete Institute) [2005]. Building code requirements for structural concrete (ACI 318–05) and commentary (ACI 318R–05). Farmington Hills, MI: American Concrete Institute.

ACI (American Concrete Institute) [2006]. Code requirements for environmental engineering concrete structures and commentary (ACI 350–06). Farmington Hills, MI: American Concrete Institute.

ASTM [2004a]. Standard test method for slake durability of shales and similar weak rock. West Conshohocken, PA: ASTM International. ASTM D–4644–87, pp. 778–780.

ASTM [2004b]. Standard test method for unconfined compressive strength of intact rock core specimens. West Conshohocken, PA: ASTM International. ASTM D–2938–95, pp. 312–314.

ASTM [2005]. Standard specification for coal fly ash and raw or calcined natural pozzolan for use in concrete. West Conshohocken, PA: ASTM International. ASTM standard C618.

ASTM [2007]. Standard specification for portland cement. West Conshohocken, PA: ASTM International. ASTM standard C150.

Barney AJ, Nair OB [1970]. In situ tests of bearing capacity of roof and floor in selected bituminous coal mines: a progress report—longwall mining. Washington, DC: U.S. Department of the Interior, U.S. Bureau of Mines, RI 7406. NTIS No. PB 193 326.

Bieniawski ZT [1992a]. Ground control. In: SME Mining Engineering Handbook. Littleton, CO: Society for Mining, Metallurgy, and Exploration, Inc., pp. 897–937.

Bieniawski ZT [1992b]. A method revisited: coal pillar strength formula based on field investigations. In: Iannacchione AT, Mark C, Repsher RC, Tuchman RJ, Jones CC, eds. Proceedings of the Workshop on Coal Pillar Mechanics and Design. Pittsburgh, PA: U.S. Department of the Interior, Bureau of Mines, IC 9315, pp. 158–165.

Chekan GJ [1985]. Design of bulkheads for controlling water in underground mines. Pittsburgh, PA: U.S. Department of Interior, Bureau of Mines, IC 9020. NTIS No. PB 85–239986.

Garrett WS, Campbell Pitt LT [1958]. Tests on an experimental underground bulkhead for high pressures. J S Afr Inst Min Metallurgy Oct.123–143.

Garrett WS, Campbell Pitt LT [1961]. Design and construction of underground bulkheads and water barriers. In: Transactions of the Seventh Commonwealth Mining and Metallurgical Congress, South African Institute of Mining and Metallurgy, pp. 1283–1301.

Harteis SP, Dolinar DR [2006]. Water and slurry bulkheads in underground coal mines: design, monitoring and safety concerns. Min Eng 58(12):41–47.

Heasley KA, Agioutantis ZG [2007]. LaModel: A boundary-element program for coal mine design. In: Mark C, Tuchman RJ, eds. Proceedings: New Technology for Ground Control in Multiple-Seam Mining. Pittsburgh, PA: U.S. Department of Health and Human Services, Public Health Service, Centers for Disease Control and Prevention, National Institute for Occupational Safety and Health, DHHS (NIOSH) Publication No. 2007–110, IC 9495, pp. 29–33.

Heasley KA, Chekan GJ [1999]. Practical boundary-element modeling for mine planning. In: Mark C, Heasley KA, Iannacchione AT, Tuchman RJ, eds. Proceedings of the Second

International Workshop on Coal Pillar Mechanics and Design. Pittsburgh, PA: U.S. Department of Health and Human Services, Public Health Service, Centers for Disease Control and Prevention, National Institute for Occupational Safety and Health, DHHS (NIOSH) Publication No. 99–114, IC 9448, pp. 73–87.

ISRM [1985]. Suggested method for determining point load strength. Int J Rock Mech Min Sci Geomech Abstr *22*:51–60.

Kendorski F [1993]. Effect of high-extraction coal mining on surface and ground water. In: Proceedings of the 12th International Conference on Ground Control in Mining. Morgantown, WV: West Virginia University, pp. 412–425.

Kendorski F [2006]. Effect of full-extraction underground mining on ground and surface waters: a 25-year retrospective. In: Proceedings of the 25th International Conference on Ground Control in Mining. Morgantown, WV: West Virginia University, pp. 425–430.

King HJ, Whittaker BN [1971]. A review of current knowledge on roadway behaviour, especially the problems on which further information is required. In: Proceedings of the Symposium on Strata Control in Roadway (1970). London: IME, pp. 73–90.

Kirkwood D, Wu K [1995]. Technical considerations for the design and construction of mine seals to withstand hydraulic heads in underground mines. SME preprint 95–100. Littleton, CO: Society for Mining, Metallurgy, and Exploration, Inc.

Mark C [2007]. Extreme multiple-seam mining in central Appalachian coalfields. In: Mark C, Tuchman RJ, eds. Proceedings: New Technology for Ground Control in Multiple-Seam Mining. Pittsburgh, PA: U.S. Department of Health and Human Services, Public Health Service, Centers for Disease Control and Prevention, National Institute for Occupational Safety and Health, DHHS (NIOSH) Publication No. 2007–110, IC 9495, pp. 55–61.

Mark C, Chase FE [1997]. Analysis of retreat mining pillar stability (ARMPS). In: Mark C, Tuchman RJ, eds. Proceedings: New Technology in Ground Control in Retreat Mining. Pittsburgh, PA: U.S. Department of Health and Human Services, Public Health Service, Centers for Disease Control and Prevention, National Institute for Occupational Safety and Health, DHHS (NIOSH) Publication No. 97–122, IC 9446, pp. 17–34.

Mark C, Molinda GM [2007]. Development and application of the coal mine roof rating (CMRR). In: Mark C, Pakalnis R, Tuchman RJ, eds. Proceedings of the International Workshop on Rock Mass Classification in Underground Mining. Pittsburgh, PA: U.S. Department of Health and Human Services, Public Health Service, Centers for Disease Control and Prevention, National Institute for Occupational Safety and Health, DHHS (NIOSH) Publication No. 2007–128, IC 9498, pp. 95–109.

Mark C, Molinda GM, Barton TM [2002]. New developments with the coal mine roof rating. In: Peng SS, Mark C, Khair AW, Heasley KA, eds. Proceedings of the 21st International Conference on Ground Control in Mining. Morgantown, WV: West Virginia University, pp. 294–301.

Merritt FS, Loftin MK, Ricketts JT [1996]. Standard handbook for civil engineers. 4th ed. McGraw-Hill.

Molinda GM, Oyler DC, Gurgenli H [2006]. Identifying moisture-sensitive roof rocks in coal mines. In: Peng SS, Mark C, Finfinger GL, Tadolini SC, Khair AW, Heasley KA, Luo Y, eds. Proceedings of the 25th International Conference on Ground Control in Mining. Morgantown, WV: West Virginia University, pp. 57–64.

MSHA and OSM [2003]. Report to Congress: responses to recommendations in the National Research Council's report "Coal waste impoundments: risks, responses, and alternatives," August 15, 2003. Appendix D: Guidance for evaluating the potential for breakthroughs from impoundments into underground mine workings and breakthrough prevention measures. U.S. Department of Labor, Mine Safety and Health Administration; and the U.S. Department of the Interior, Office of Surface Mining, Reclamation, and Enforcement, Appendix D, pp. 41–45.

NIOSH [2008a]. NIOSH mining software: Analysis of Retreat Mining Pillar Stability (ARMPS). [http://www.cdc.gov/NIOSH/Mining/products/product6.htm]. Date accessed: February 2008.

NIOSH [2008b]. NIOSH mining software: stress and displacement calculations (LaModel). [http://www.cdc.gov/niosh/mining/products/product54.htm]. Date accessed: February 2008.

Park R, Paulay T [1975]. Reinforced concrete structures. New York: John Wiley and Sons, Inc.

Peng SS [1986]. Coal mine ground control. 2nd ed. New York: John Wiley and Sons, Inc.

Pytel W [1994]. On pillar design for weak floor strata conditions. In: Proceedings of the Fifth Conference on Ground Control in Midwest U.S. Coal Mines (Collinsville, IL, June 27–30, 1994), pp. 88–110.

Ross T, Klobuka L, Vandergrift T, Choi J [1998]. Analysis of panel stability for post-mining slurry injection. In: Proceedings of the 17th International Conference on Ground Control in Mining. Morgantown, WV: West Virginia University, pp. 284–292.

Rusnak J, Mark C [2000]. Using the point load test to determine the uniaxial compressive strength of coal measure rock. In: Peng SS, Mark C, eds. Proceedings of the 19th International Conference on Ground Control in Mining. Morgantown, WV: West Virginia University, pp. 362–371.

Sherard JL, Decker RS, eds. [1977]. Dispersive clays, related piping, and erosion in geotechnical projects. STP 623. West Conshohocken, PA: ASTM International.

Speck R [1981]. The influence of certain geologic and geotechnical factors on coal mine floor stability: a case study. In: Proceedings of the First Conference on Ground Control in Mining. Morgantown, WV: West Virginia University, pp. 44–49.

Su D, Scandrol R, Hasenfus G [1993]. Development and evaluation of a floor-bearing capacity test apparatus. In: Proceedings of the 12th International Conference on Ground Control in Mining. Morgantown, WV: West Virginia University, pp. 357–365.

Timoshenko S, Woinowsky-Kreiger S [1959]. Theory of plates and shells. 2nd ed. McGraw-Hill Publishing Co.

Tulanowski R, Kirkwood D, Gardner G [1993]. Non-injury water inundation, Meigs No. 31 Mine (I.D. No. 33–01172), Southern Ohio Coal Company, Langsville, Meigs County, Ohio. Arlington, VA: U.S. Department of Labor, Mine Safety and Health Administration.

Unrug K [1997]. Weatherability test of rocks for underground mines. In: Proceedings of the 16th International Conference on Ground Control in Mining. Morgantown, WV: West Virginia University, pp. 259–266.

U.S. Bureau of Reclamation [1975]. Concrete manual. 8th ed. Washington, DC: U.S. Department of the Interior, Bureau of Reclamation.

Winter G, Nilson A [1979]. Design of concrete structures. 9th ed. McGraw-Hill Book Co.

Wu K, Owens H, Fredland J [2003]. MSHA's review of impoundment plans. SME preprint No. 03–099. Littleton, CO: Society for Mining, Metallurgy, and Exploration, Inc.

Young W [1989]. Roark's formulas for stress and strain. 6th ed. New York: McGraw-Hill, Inc.

APPENDIX A.—ADDITIONAL GUIDANCE FOR MAPS AND DRAWINGS

All maps and drawings submitted in the permit package should:

- Be of sufficient scale and font size to adequately detail the information being conveyed. Information that is illegible or unclear could result in return of the permit application for clarification or corrections.
- Contain a legend detailing symbols, shading, and color representations, if applicable.
- Contain a title block that indicates the title of the drawing, scale, mine or operation name, federal and state identification numbers, drawing number, name of consulting or engineering firm if applicable, date, and location of the operation.
- Be certified by a professional engineer registered in the state in which the operation is located.

The following is a list of maps and drawings that must be submitted in the permit application, along with information requirements. Depending on the size of the operation and the size of the fluid retention system, some of the maps and drawings may be combined.

Impoundment Map

- Provide a map highlighting the entire impoundment area. Indicate the mine works to be inundated and the anticipated shoreline at the maximum anticipated fluid level.
- Show the proposed location of the bulkhead structure(s).
- Using the mine floor elevations, provide contour lines for the impoundment area not to exceed 5-ft intervals.

Bulkhead Structure Map and/or Drawing(s)

- Provide a horizontal and vertical cross-section of the proposed location(s) with roof and floor elevations.
- Include dimensions of each mine entry with details for notching the roof, ribs, and floor, if required.
- Pipes or other conduits passing through the bulkhead structure must be designated on this drawing. Include pipe function, size(s), and pressure rating, and provide details such as antiseep collars for preventing fluid flow between the pipe and bulkhead structure.
- Indicate proposed location of pressure gauges, transducers, flow gauges, and other devices used to monitor the fluid level and flow into and out of the fluid retention structure.
- Detail the type, spacing, and location(s) of additional ground control measures to be installed. Include planned strata grouting.
- Detail measures taken to reduce leakage between the strata and bulkhead structure.
- Reference detailed drawings, if needed, to convey additional information.

Affected Area Map

It is important to detail the underground and surface areas that could become inundated if the proposed bulkhead system fails. For this purpose, a mine map should be submitted that details the complete underground workings associated with that operation, including sealed areas and adjacent mine workings within the same seam that are physically connected to the operation (even if separated by a seal or bulkhead). Requirements include the following:

- Use a scale suitable to convey the extent of the mine works that would be inundated if a bulkhead or system failure occurs.
- Include mine floor contours at no less than 10-ft intervals.
- Identify mine works where the fluid will roof out, areas that are flooded but not roofed, and unaffected areas.
- Identify all ventilation seals that could be exposed to head pressure, and highlight those that could be exposed to pressures greater than their rated explosive pressure.
- Identify shafts, slopes, and other openings from the surface to underground workings that would be affected.
- Identify main power distribution equipment that would be affected.

If the surface area could be impacted by a bulkhead system failure, a surface area map should also be included. Requirements include the following:

- Indicate the surface openings that could act as a conduit for the fluid to reach the surface.
- Indicate the surface area permitted by the mining operation.
- Indicate the anticipated fluid flow path from the impoundment to the point it reaches the surface, then from the surface to the discharge point into a receiving stream or until it leaves the permit area.
- Include surface contours at no less than 10-ft intervals.

Adjacent Mine Works Map

A complete set of mine maps should be submitted that details all adjacent mine works within the same mining horizon and any mine works above or below the impoundment if located within at least 1,000 ft of the perimeter. Two situations must be considered. Will water from the adjacent works flow into the planned impoundment, or will water from the planned impoundment flow into the adjacent works? In most mining operations, mining in horizons below the impoundment will not create a flow into the impoundment. However, due to the dip of a seam, if sections of a flooded mine below the impoundment are higher in elevation than the impoundment, the head pressure from the workings below can be sufficient to allow an inflow of fluid from the lower works to the impoundment. Requirements include the following:

- Overlay and underlay contour maps indicating the location and extent of mine workings located within at least a 1,000-ft perimeter of the impoundment. This will include mining in horizons above, below, and within the same seam as the proposed impoundment. More than one mining horizon can be indicated on a map, but the horizons must be easily distinguishable.

46

- Indicate known areas of impounded water in other mining horizons.
- Give details for any boreholes or other openings that could connect the impoundment with adjacent seams.
- Note interburden distances between the proposed fluid retention impoundment and overlying and underlying mine works.

Surface Features Map

The map should locate all surface water sources that could impact the underground fluid retention system. It should overlay the proposed underground impoundment area with the surface topography map, which identifies all sources of surface water including ponds, streams, lakes, rivers, and any other surface impoundments. Requirements include the following:

- The map should extend at least 1,000 ft beyond the outer perimeter of the proposed underground impoundment.
- Include surface and mine seam contours.
- Identify all surface water sources.
- Identify any structures that could act as a conduit for fluid to flow from the surface to the underground impoundment.

APPENDIX B.—SAMPLE BULKHEAD INSPECTION SHEET

Examiner: _____   Shift: 1   2   3

Date: _____

	Time	Pressure	% O_2	% CH_4	CO ppm	Leakage (gpm)
Bulkhead No. 1						
Bulkhead No. 2						
Bulkhead No. 3						
Bulkhead No. 4						

Condition of bulkhead structures:
(Note any changes in physical condition, deflection, and signs of stress.)

Roof and rib observations:
(Note any sloughing or other changes.)

Leakage observations:
(Note any changes or new leakage locations.)

Other conditions observed:

_____
Shift Foreman

_____   _____
Mine Foreman   **Superintendent**

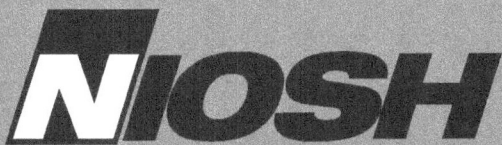

Delivering on the Nation's promise:
safety and health at work for all people
through research and prevention

To receive NIOSH documents or more information about
occupational safety and health topics, contact NIOSH at

1–800–CDC–INFO (1–800–232–4636)
TTY: 1–888–232–6348
e-mail: cdcinfo@cdc.gov

or visit the NIOSH Web site at **www.cdc.gov/niosh.**

For a monthly update on news at NIOSH, subscribe to
NIOSH *eNews* by visiting **www.cdc.gov/niosh/eNews.**

DHHS (NIOSH) Publication No. 2008–134

SAFER • HEALTHIER • PEOPLE™

www.ingramcontent.com/pod-product-compliance
Lightning Source LLC
Chambersburg PA
CBHW080910290526
45795CB00007BA/2483